The
Fat Flush
Fitness
Plan

Also by Ann Louise Gittleman:

The Fat Flush Plan
The Fat Flush Cookbook
The Fat Flush Journal and Shopping Guide
The Complete Fat Flush Program
Ann Louise Gittleman's Guide to the 40–30–30 Phenomenon
Before the Change
Beyond Pritikin
Eat Fat, Lose Weight
Eat Fat, Lose Weight Cookbook
Get the Salt Out
Get the Sugar Out
Guess What Came to Dinner?
How to Stay Young & Healthy
The Living Beauty Detox Program
Super Nutrition for Men
Super Nutrition for Menopause
Super Nutrition for Women
Why Am I Always So Tired?
Your Body Knows Best

Also by Joanie Greggains:

Fit Happens

The
Fat Flush
Fitness
Plan

ANN LOUISE GITTLEMAN M.S., C.N.S.
and
JOANIE GREGGAINS

McGraw-Hill

New York / Chicago / San Francisco / Lisbon / London
Madrid / Mexico City / Milan / New Delhi / San Juan
Seoul / Singapore / Sydney / Toronto

The **McGraw·Hill** Companies

To men and women everywhere

who long for a fresh and

unique fitness approach

Library of Congress Cataloging-in-Publication Data
Gittleman, Ann Louise. The fat flush fitness plan / By Ann Louise Gittleman and
Joanie Greggains.—1st ed.
    p. cm.
Includes index.
 ISBN 0-07-142312-5 (hbk. : alk. paper)
 1. Reducing exercises. 2. Exercise for women. 3. Physical fitness
for women. 4. Cellulite. I. Greggains, Joanie. II. Title.
 RA781.6.G55 2004
 613.7'1—dc22

                                                                    2003015873

34567890 DOC/DOC 09876543

ISBN 0-07-142312-5

Printed and bound by RR Donnelley.

This book is for educational purposes. It is not intended as a substitute for individual fitness, health,
and medical advice. Please consult a qualified health care professional for individual health and
medical advice. Neither McGraw-Hill nor the authors shall have any responsibility for any adverse effects
arising directly or indirectly as a result of the information provided in this book.

McGraw-Hill books are available at special quantity discounts to use as premiums and sales promotions,
or for use in corporate training programs. For more information, please write to the Director of Special
Sales, Professional Publishing, McGraw-Hill, Two Penn Plaza, New York, NY 10121-2298. Or contact your
local bookstore.

Contents

Preface

*The real voyage of discovery consists not in seeking new landscapes,
but in having new eyes.*

— MARCEL PROUST

What If It's All Been a Big, Fat Lie?

That's the title of a landmark article in the *New York Times* questioning what up to now has been the reigning orthodoxy in U.S. diet and nutrition. "Low-fat weight-loss diets have proved . . . to be dismal failures," writes Gary Taubes in the July 7, 2002, article.[1] As scientists from the U.S. Department of Agriculture to the Harvard School of Public Health now realize, eliminating fat from our diets does not reduce the rate of heart disease—but it has helped increase the rate of obesity. Between 50 and 80 percent of the U.S. population is overweight,[2] in part because their diets are deficient in omega-3 and omega-6 polyunsaturated fats that actually help your body metabolize fat.

But low-fat diets aren't the only culprit in today's skyrocketing obesity statistics. If you are concerned about weight gain or weight retention, you may be surprised to learn that the culprits may also include stress, lack of sleep, and, very possibly, excess exercise.

That's right. Too much exercise can actually make it harder for you to lose weight. Although it's true that many Americans don't exercise enough, it's also true that some exercise too much. Overexercise—especially combined with insufficient sleep, excessive stress, and poor eating habits—can actually send your body into survival mode, raising your levels of cortisol and other stress-related hormones and instructing your body to hold onto its fat.

There is an alternative to the world of unbalanced diet and exercise plans—and this is it. My work as a nutritionist has taken me on an incredible journey over the past fifteen years, from work at the Pritikin Center—a major advocate of low-fat diets—to a gradual disillusioment with their approach and the ongoing evolution of mine. When I first published *Beyond Pritikin* in 1988, I was just starting to grasp the principles on which all my subsequent work has been based: detoxifying and cleansing the liver, combating the excess production of insulin, and taking a holistic, nurturing approach to women's bodies, supporting their overall health as a crucial element in enabling them to lose weight. At that point, I had created only a two-week version of the Fat Flush Plan. By the time I published *The Fat Flush Plan*, I had developed a lifelong program that empowers women to lose weight through detoxification, cleansing, balanced nutrition, and the creation of a healthy lifestyle.

I went on to publish *The Fat Flush Cookbook* and *The Fat Flush Journal and Shopping Guide*, and I founded the Fatflush.com Forum in 2003 to offer ongoing support to women and men seeking to maintain this healthy approach for the rest of their lives. But I sensed that a major element was still missing. Although there were some elements of a fitness program in *The Fat Flush Plan*, many of my readers and Internet community members wanted a more structured fitness program. They wanted to know what kinds of exercise would support their new way of eating, their new respect and love for their bodies, their new holistic approach to health. They wanted to be sure that if they lost large amounts of weight, their skin would stay toned and firm. And, like most women in our society, they wanted to target their hips, thighs, abs, arms, and derrieres, becoming slimmer and more shapely as they lost pounds and inches.

Enter Joanie Greggains, a San Francisco-based fitness expert who has been a pioneering voice for balance in exercise. From the first, Joanie has pointed out that a balanced exercise program combining cardiovascular activities with strength training and stretching is far more effective for weight loss and body shaping than a punishing exercise program where the body is constantly under stress to perform and never has time to repair, a type of exercise that can lead to weight gain, fatigue, and injury.

I first met Joanie when she invited me to be a guest on her KGO Radio talk show in San Francisco in 1992. Joanie had picked up on my work right away, and as my approach to eating has evolved, Joanie has shared it with the thousands of women who enroll in her fit camps, in which about a dozen women meet once a week for four weeks to learn about diet, exercise, and other healthy lifestyle choices based on fact, not fiction.

Joanie is the author of two important fitness books, *Total Body Shape Up* and *Fit Happens*, as well as the producer and star of some fifteen exercise videos, for which she's won two gold record awards, nine gold video-casettes, and six platinum cassettes. She was the host and star of *Morning Stretch*, a syndicated half-hour TV exercise show that ran in over 100 markets through the 1990s, and she continues to be a sought after speaker on health and fitness.

But it wasn't her star power that attracted me most, or the strong personal friendship that the two of us developed over the years. It wasn't even the fact that, through more than a decade of recommending the Fat Flush eating plan to her fit camp members, Joanie had lots of hands-on experience observing women on my eating plan, giving her a solid base of knowledge with which to design a companion fitness program.

These things were important. But even more important was the fact that, like me, Joanie was something of a maverick, going up against the exercise establishment just as I had taken on the diet world. During the years when I was arguing that a low-fat diet actually creates weight gain, fatigue, sugar cravings, and other serious problems, Joanie was explaining that overexercise and high-impact fitness programs were actually creating health problems for women, sabotaging their weight loss efforts and ultimately sapping their energy. Just as I was trying to create an eating plan that would nurture every woman's body, mind, and spirit, so was Joanie working toward an approach to exercise designed to work with the body, not against it.

For both of us, the Fat Flush approach has become the exciting culmination of our efforts, separately and together. We've worked closely to create *The Fat Flush Fitness Plan*, based on a single basic biological premise: cleansing the liver and the lymphatic system is absolutely crucial for physical health, weight loss, and an overall sense of well-being. Women who detox their livers and get their lymph flowing—two goals that these eating and fitness plans are perfectly designed to do—notice that they have clear, glowing skin; firm, toned bodies; and virtually unbounded reserves of energy. As an added bonus, this approach to eating and fitness seems also to make cellulite less visible—at least, that's what hundreds of women who've tried our plan have told us.

Although the Fat Flush Fitness Plan has been designed to support the Fat Flush eating plan, you can just buy this book and start exercising. I promise that you'll feel better, look better, and astound your friends, family, coworkers, and loved ones with the amazing levels of energy you acquire in just a few days. If you're intrigued by this approach, however, I urge you to pick up a copy of *The Fat Flush Plan* as well, so that you can try the eating plan along with the fitness plan. You'll discover that it is an exponentially faster way of making progress toward your weight loss and fitness goals, reshaping your body even as you boost your mental focus, calm your emotions, release your stress, and discover levels of energy and serenity that you could only dream about before.

I know it sounds like I'm exaggerating. But I'm not. Both Joanie and I have seen this plan work for literally thousands of women—and for ourselves as well. So welcome to the Fat Flush community. I look forward to sharing the fruits of our labors with you.

ANN LOUISE GITTLEMAN

Acknowledgments

To my mother and father, Edith and Arthur, I am very blessed to have you as parents. Thank you for instilling in me a strong New England work ethic and teaching me—by being a living example of the wisdom of the Talmud—that the world is based upon three things: work, study, and deeds of loving kindness. You have been the most steadfast cheering section in my life and always made me feel I could do and achieve anything. It is truly an honor to be your daughter.

To my brother Stuart, thanks for your unerring support throughout the years and thanks for growing into such a fine leader and directing the course of First Lady of Nutrition, Inc. Producers, editors, and public relations/marketing executives are always so impressed with your "style" and "finesse." You have no idea how many offers I receive for your services.

To my sister-in-law Sandra, you are a powerful presence rooting us on from backstage. You are doing such a magnificent job in raising Isaac and Daniel and mentoring Shira. Thank you for everything you do with such a loving and devoted heart. I am especially grateful for your understanding when Stuart has to be on the road with me for long stretches.

I couldn't have done this without Joanie Greggains. Her enthusiasm, sparkle, expertise, and insight have inspired me in so many ways. I am so thankful to have coauthored this book with her.

To Linda, Mary, Carol L, Sue, Jackie, Barbara, Kathy, and Martha: Your commitment and devotion to the Fat Flush messaging boards on the Forum and ivillage touches me very deeply. Together we can and have made such a difference in the quality of so many individuals' lives. Your support morning, noon, and night is so appreciated and valued.

Thank you to Grant and Renee Magan for assisting me in making my home environment organized and clean. You have helped to create a haven of regeneration and rejuvenation for my body, mind, and spirit in so many ways.

To J. Lynne Dodson and Jonny Bowden whose initial creative efforts were so formative in the evolution of this manuscript.

Heartfelt thanks and acknowledgment goes to Rachel Krantz who assisted in transforming our ideas and inspiration into concrete fitness advice. You came on board at the last minute (literally) and proved your worth a thousand times over. You conveyed our passion and our personalities. May we have an opportunity in the very near future to work together again.

To the team at McGraw Hill—from Philip Ruppel, our steadfast publisher to Nancy Hancock, our absolutely brilliant editor to Meg Leder, Nancy's irreplaceable assistant, to Ann Pryor, our devoted public relations manager to Lynda Luppino, our supportive marketing director. Our editor, Rena Copperman was so committed to this project and gave of her time above and beyond the call of duty.

Thank you to Marsha Cohen for her beautiful interior book design and to Tom Lau for the lovely cover design. My heartfelt gratitude to Bob Tinnon for executing the design and turning it into the pages you are about to read.

I would also like to acknowledge Cindy Renshaw, Joanie's personal assistant, who exemplifies the gold standard in personal assistanthood.

Finally, my most sincere thanks to JWT, my life partner, whose patience and love were tested during this writing process but who nevertheless managed to build the most beautiful new home for both of us on the Spokane River. Thanks for providing me with a healing haven.

ANN LOUISE GITTLEMAN

No one truly writes a book alone. I'd like to thank the following people for their support, encouragement, and advice that made this book possible.

First of all, Ann Louise Gittleman, for believing in me; my assistant Cindy Renshaw, as always, invaluable; Nancy Hancock, editor extraordinaire; Meg Leder, always helpful; Rachel Krantz, word master; Rena Copperman, "The Fixer," able to pull it all together without every losing her sense of humor; Caren Alpert, photographer, for making it all work; and Meridian Sports Clubs, Rolling Hills, Novato, California. Owner Chuck Grieve and his wonderful staff—Mary Beth Bradley, Patty Fields, and Alison Abbott—provided the perfect background for our photographs.

Special thanks to my husband, Robert McDonald, for his love, support, and for "holding down the fort," which made it possible for me to do this book.

Thank you to Jeannette Boudreau, Esquire; Bill Kirby, Sylvie DeSegur, and Rose Cologne for their professional help; and to my mentors, Philip Dubrow (both in business and in life) and Jim Dunbar (best broadcaster and Renaissance man).

For professional guidance, I'd like to acknowledge Dr. James Garrick, Dr. Donald Chu, Dr. George Markle, Dr. Brunno Ristow, Dr. Laurie Green, Dr. Karl Knopf, Dr. Richard Shames, Dr. Elson Haas, Dr. Ronald Smialowicz, Dr. James Farrell, Debra Francesconi, R.N., and Michael Machado.

Special thanks to my girlfriends, Parry Garrett and Melanie Morgan; Joan Cresci; Sheila Collins (the Godmother; Sean Galvin (dignity and grace always); Suzie Nails; Jack and Elaine LaLanne; Maury Povich; my fabulous 7:30 A.M. exercise class; and all my Fit Campers, with a special thanks to Loretta Bracco, Linda Zider, Bev Giraudo, and Patricia Johnson for the joy they brought to the photos in this book.

Let the journey begin.

JOANIE GREGGAINS

Introduction

We can do anything we want as long as we stick to it long enough.

—HELEN KELLER

As a fitness professional with a lifelong interest in making people healthier, fitter, and happier, I've always been interested in nutrition. But for many years, I was frustrated with the information I was getting from the diet establishment. As a nationally known radio talk show host, I had the opportunity to interview just about everyone in the nutrition and diet field—but frankly, their ideas just didn't make sense to me. I could see for myself-from the thousands of women I worked with each year—that their orthodoxy of high carbs, low fat, and an overemphasis on calorie counting simply wasn't effective for many women. In fact, for many of my clients, that approach was an outright disaster.

When I first read the original version of the Fat Flush Plan in Ann Louise's 1988 book *Beyond Pritikin*, I knew I was on to something special. Here was a woman who'd actually been in the trenches, at the Pritikin Center itself, the very bastion of low-fat orthodoxy. When she blew the whistle on this approach, her response was based on years of experience with thousands of clients. She was saying out loud something I'd suspected for years: the high-carb, low-fat approach just didn't work.

I was so impressed with what I read that I tried the Fat Flush program myself. For the first time in my life—and remember, I'd been exercising up a storm since I was a teenager—those five extra pounds that I'd never been able to shake actually dropped off without effort, something that had not happened with any eating plan I'd ever tried. I invited Ann Louise onto my radio show, and soon she became a regular guest—and a friend.

As Ann Louise points out in her Preface, we were partly drawn together by our "maverick" status. While Ann Louise was taking on the low-fat dogma, I was questioning aerobics orthodoxy, which in the 1980s and early 1990s advocated high-impact programs that left women feeling stressed, exhausted, and overworked. Sure, it *felt* like you had accomplished something when your body was pushed that hard. But in the end, women who went that route weren't really losing all the weight they wanted to. A high-impact exercise program was somewhat effective for the cardiovascular system. But it didn't do much for hip, thigh, and belly fat, and it seemed useless in releasing "false fat" or bloat—the water retention that, as Ann Louise explains in *The Fat Flush Plan*, can cause you to swell up 10 to 15 pounds or one to two dress sizes simply because your lower body tissues are clinging desperately to excess fluids due to a poor diet, hormonal imbalance, or medications.[1]

I had already discovered that my clients who undertook a more balanced program of low-impact aerobics, weight training, and proper stretching were able to reshape their lower bodies as well. But they still seemed to lack the boundless reserves of energy I thought my exercise program would provide, and some were still bothered with water retention and "belly bloat."

When I recommended that my clients try Ann Louise's eating plan in addition to my fitness program, however, I noticed a dramatic shift. Suddenly, just as I myself had found, they were losing the extra belly fat that had always plagued them, their bodies were taking on a new sleek, toned level of fitness, and their skin was clear and glowing as it had never been before. Working with Ann Louise on the biology behind her work and mine, we discovered that the key was in cleansing the liver and the lymphatic system, an approach that is best accomplished through a combined eating and fitness program.

Ann Louise and I had both noticed, too, that stress, lack of sleep, and a disregard for one's own emotional life were not only unpleasant experiences for most women but were actual factors in weight gain and weight retention. We were both looking for approaches to diet and fitness that allowed women to honor themselves and their feelings, to get the deep sleep they needed, and to respect their emotional and physical boundaries. I'd always felt instinctively that these were important elements in a healthy life, but only when I met Ann Louise did I come to realize that they were more than simply "extras"—they are the very foundation of our physical well-being. It sounds dramatic, but it's true: If you're not sleeping enough, if you're overstressed and undernourished—either physically or emotionally—you're going to find it nearly impossible to lose weight. If you take proper care of yourself, resting, sleeping, and paying attention to your thoughts, feelings, and spiritual needs, you'll be amazed how the fat melts away.

We explain the biology for all this in Chapter 1, so I won't go into it again here. I'll only add that one more source of stress for many women these days is lack of community. A number of recent studies suggest that isolation can actually be detrimental to our health, while friendship, companionship, and community support can add years to our lives.[2] One of the benefits of adopting the Fat Flush approach to eating and fitness is your opportunity to join the Fat Flush community by participating in the fatflush.com Web site. Certainly, my friendship with Ann Louise has been an enormous source of support and health for me. It's exciting to see that over a decade of professional and personal association has resulted in a book that integrates each of our life's work: a holistic approach to health and fitness that will improve your body, mind, and spirit beyond your wildest dreams.

JOANIE GREGGAINS

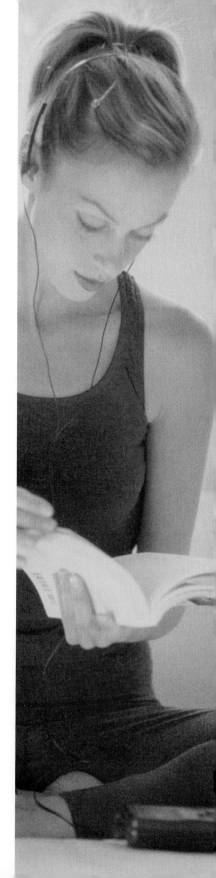

1

The Surprising Truth About Exercise and Weight Loss

We live in a world of problems which can no longer be solved by the level of thinking which created them.

—ALBERT EINSTEIN

Emily was a thirty-five-year-old mother of two who also worked full-time as an emergency room nurse. She was constantly on the go, caring for her children, her patients, her husband—everyone but herself. Although Emily protested that she barely ate two meals a day, let alone three, and never allowed herself the sweet snacks she craved, she was constantly fighting an extra 10 or 15 pounds of fat around her hips, as well as struggling with low energy, a short temper, and the frustrating sense that she was too busy to enjoy herself. "I work so hard and do so much," Emily told Joanie tearfully, "you'd think all that activity would at least *burn off some calories!*"

Madison was a self-described "exercise fanatic." A twenty-two-year-old former ballet student, she was now back in school with the goal of becoming a physical therapist. Despite her studies, she managed

1

to run 5 miles a day, take two ballet classes a week, and on the weekends, for fun, she played a little tennis. She also followed a relatively strict low-calorie, low-fat diet, fighting her perpetual hunger pangs with regular infusions of coffee and an occasional cigarette. Although she considered herself "basically a cheerful person," Madison had been taking the antidepressant Paxil for about a year. Because she'd experienced wildly irregular menstrual periods ever since she started menstruating, her gynecologist had also put her on birth control pills. Despite her regular exercise and stringent diet, Madison was plagued by midriff fat that had bothered her throughout her career as a dancer. "If I can't get rid of it now, at my age," she asked Ann Louise, "what will I do when I get older?"

Kate had never liked exercise, and it was only sheer desperation after a doctor's warning that drove her to one of Joanie's fit camps. A short, round woman in her late fifties, Kate explained that her weight had simply climbed up over the years, particularly after each of her three pregnancies—so that now she was at least 35 pounds overweight. She'd been an off-and-on dieter for years, and became concerned that if a diet ever did work, she'd be facing huge, ugly flaps of skin hanging off her arms and neck. Meanwhile, her doctor had put her on Lipitor for her rising cholesterol. Kate loved her work as a financial analyst, but she admitted that she often went for weeks on fewer than six hours of sleep a night. "I don't know when I'll find time to exercise," she told Joanie briskly, "but it's doctor's orders, so let's get started!"

Emily, Madison, and Kate are composite portraits of the women that we meet every day, women seeking nutritional counseling, exercise coaching, or both. We became committed to developing an integrated diet and exercise plan that enhanced the results of each component. Through our work with thousands of women who have lost both pounds and inches, we came up with the Fat Flush fitness program, an approach to exercise specifically designed to target the hidden reasons that women have trouble losing weight.

When followed along with the Fat Flush eating plan, the Fat Flush Fitness Plan can help you achieve the following goals:

- weight loss
- the ability to rid yourself of unwanted tummy fat
- loss of inches at your hips, waist, and thighs
- tightened-up muscles for improved skin tone, including the upper arms
- a higher rear and firmer buttocks
- enhanced lean muscle mass
- stronger connective tissue, making your entire body more limber and flexible
- significant reduction in the appearance of cellulite

If you eat and exercise the Fat Flush way, you'll discover that you have almost miraculous new reserves of energy, even as you lose weight and reshape your body. That's because both the diet and the exercise plan are based on a solid understanding of human anatomy—and of women's bodies in particular.

Of course, in the process, you may have to revise a few long-held assumptions about how your body works and what it needs. Through years of working with women, both of us have become accustomed to the raised eyebrows, skeptical looks, and downright challenges to the following basic principles that underlie the Fat Flush system:

1. Detoxifying your liver is crucial to losing unwanted weight.
2. Stimulating the lymphatic system is the key to effective exercise and weight loss.

Check with Your Doctor
Exercise is terrific—but not everyone is ready to jump right into a new fitness regimen. We urge you to talk to your physician or health care practitioner before you start the Fat Flush Fitness Plan if you're not already doing regular exercise and if

- you're a woman over age fifty or a man over forty and you haven't had a physical exam in over two years.

- you've got an unstable medical condition, such as uncontrolled high blood pressure or diabetes.

- you're pregnant or have just had a baby (and see Chapter 8 for a modified plan when you do start exercising).

- you smoke.

- you have joint problems or osteoporosis.

- you have cuts or wounds that are slow to heal.

- you are significantly overweight (100 pounds or more over what your doctor considers a healthy weight).

- you have a family history of heart disease or stroke.

3. Stress—including excessive exercise and lack of sleep—is probably the most insidious weight gain factor among U.S. women today.

Let's take a closer look at each one of these principles—each based on years of research, study, and working with thousands of women.

The Basic Principles of the Fat Flush System

Detoxifying Your Liver Is Crucial to Losing Unwanted Weight

Ann Louise's book, *The Fat Flush Plan*, presents the discoveries that laid the foundation for the Fat Flush diet and exercise plan.[1]

The liver has two major functions: to detoxify the blood and to break down fat. A healthy, high-functioning liver breaks down fat efficiently, provided that we supply it with fat-metabolizing nutrients and liver-supporting herbs and enzymes. Unfortunately, most of our livers are simply overstressed. These organs were designed to remove the toxins that occur naturally in our bodies, such as the ammonia that forms when protein is metabolized. But our poor livers are now doing double, triple, and even quadruple duty purifying the toxins we deliberately invite into our systems—alcohol, caffeine, trans fats (margarine, vegetable shortening, and fried foods), sugars and sweeteners, and drugs, including prescription medications, hormones, legal over-the-counter medicines—especially Tylenol or any drug containing acetaminophen—and some herbal/nutritional supplements, such as valerian, pennyroyal, ephedra (*ma huang*), high-dose vitamin A, and others. As if that weren't enough, our livers must also filter out the air pollution, additives, preservatives, toxic fumes, and chemicals or parasites in our tap water (think chlorine, fluoride, and giardia) that assault most of us every day.

When the liver is overloaded, it dumps the toxins into the bile. The thick, viscous bile that results cannot properly emulsify fat—and that little bulge at your waistline is the result.

Given how hard we make them work, no wonder our livers can't metabolize fat properly! Many years ago, when Ann Louise first began directing her clients to consume liver-supporting foods—such as eggs (especially the yolks) and the juice of fresh lemons squeezed in hot water—she noticed a remarkable drop in weight even when the rest of her clients' diet and exercise patterns remained the same. Freeing up your liver to do its job might be the single most important step you'll ever take in improving your overall health and achieving your weight loss goals.

Both Madison and Kate were surprised to learn that medications they had considered relatively harmless—Paxil, birth control pills, and Lipitor—could be stressing their livers and interfering with their attempts at weight loss. Madison knew that caffeine and tobacco were not the healthiest of substances, but she was astonished to learn that her daily mugs of coffee and regular cigarette smoking—which she'd always seen as weight loss aids—were actually setting the stage for excess fat deposition. And all three women were intrigued—yet somewhat skeptical—at the idea that cutting back on liver stressors might endow them with more energy.

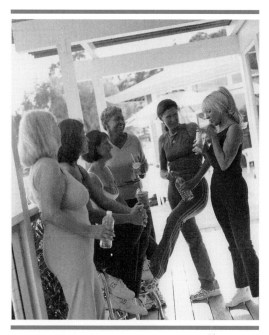

Over the years, Ann Louise developed a three-phase Fat Flush eating plan, with the first stage focusing on detoxification and support of the liver. She found that this focus on the liver could produce extraordinary weight loss results, even after only two weeks. (Check with your doctor before discontinuing or modifying the dosage of any prescription medication.)

But although this detox process ultimately leads to high energy levels, better hormonal balance, glowing skin, improved digestion, a healthier cadiovascular system, and an enhanced immune system, it can be tiring at first. The oil-soluble toxins that barrage us in twenty-first-century America are deposited in body fat, insulating them from the rest of our systems. As body fat begins to melt away, we're exposed to these toxins as they're recirculated in the system, which can sometimes cause minor fatigue and/or discomfort. Ann Louise has carefully constructed the Fat Flush eating plan and her fiber-rich "Long Life Cocktail" to mitigate these effects—but the first two weeks on her eating plan can sometimes be a bit tiring, so we'd like you to take it easy.

Moreover, although cutting out the "artificial highs" of sugar and caffeine does eventually provide you with new levels of energy, your initial reaction to withdrawing from these addictive substances can also be tiring and uncomfortable. So the Fat Flush fitness program has its own phase 1, allowing your body to rest, recuperate, and readjust as your liver recovers its health. But rest assured: as we lessen the toxic load, your body will be doing the job it was always intended to do—and we'll give you all the nutritional support you will need during this process.

Tips for Making Time to Work Out

- **Make a contract with yourself.** If you're really serious about making a change, doing something good for yourself, and taking charge of your health, then make a commitment. There's always time to do the things that are really important to us—so your first step is to decide that your health is important to you. In order to be a success at your fitness program, you need to challenge yourself to make an active, ironclad commitment to it. Once you've made this commitment, you'll be surprised at how much time suddenly becomes available. In fact, we suggest making a formal promise to yourself, in writing (see page 40 toward the end of Chapter 2 for a sample pledge that you can use as a model).

- **Turn off the phone.** There's nothing that disrupts our lives more consistently and insistently than the telephone. Don't let Ma Bell interfere with *your* workout! Turn off your home phone. Turn down the volume on your answering machine. And leave your cell phone at home if you go out for a walk. This is your time, and you have to make that clear both to yourself and the other people in your life.

- **Be good to yourself.** Honestly, if you haven't been exercising regularly, you haven't been very good to yourself. Now is your chance to turn all that around. One way to get started is to stop considering your workout a punishment and start making it a treat. Challenge yourself to find ways that you can make your workout more fun. How about adding music? Would you enjoy rebounding more if you could watch TV or a rebounding DVD/video while you bounced? What if you started each workout by rubbing a little scented lotion over your arms and legs, to remind yourself of how much you love your body and how grateful you are to your muscles for exerting themselves? Have you chosen an exercise outfit whose colors and textures make you happy? Maybe you'd get a little pleasure out of some extra soft socks. Think of something—or a variety of things—you could do to associate pleasure with your workout time.

- **Encourage yourself.** Become your own best friend—and your own toughest coach. Buy products that will motivate you to work out, such as a heart rate monitor to see how fast your heart is beating when you start the Fat Flush Fitness Plan—and then to track how your heart rate falls as you get into shape. (We've listed some consumer information in Chapter 10 of this book.) Monitoring your improvement with a heart rate monitor can be a kind of instant gratification that keeps you motivated. Keeping a workout journal is also helpful. Something about recording your day's workout reminds you that you've accomplished something, simply by showing up and doing what you've promised yourself to do. Looking back over your journal can also be an exciting way of tracking your progress.

- Respect your own rhythms. For this program to work, you need to know what works for you—and then be 100 percent committed to making sure you've got it. Finding the right times and rhythms for exercise means that you've got a no-excuse zero-tolerance exercise program in place that you will definitely fulfill. Some people prefer to exercise first thing in the morning. Others do much better in the late afternoon or early evening, when vigorous exercise can be a terrific way to release all the accumulated stress of the day. Likewise, some people love a set routine—"I exercise every single day at 8 A.M. rain or shine"—while other people thrive on variety. Perhaps you already know the approach that works for you, or maybe you'll need to experiment a little as you start this new regimen. Either way, start from a place of respect for your own rhythms and preferences, and craft your exercise plan accordingly.

- Be honest with yourself. Too many of us lie to ourselves, insisting that we'll start exercising "someday" without ever really taking responsibility for the fact that we haven't done it—and aren't likely to do it. If you really don't want to exercise, put down this book and resign yourself to an unhealthy life and an uncomfortable old age. If you are really ready to get moving, then make a commitment and get started.

- Remember, you only get one body—but that body will come through for you if you let it! Stop waiting for a miracle and start moving! In the time it's taken you to come up with three reasons you're too busy to exercise, you could have walked a brisk mile and done a little stretching. As we get older, it's easy to give in to the myth that aging means becoming less active, less flexible, and ultimately less capable. But it really doesn't have to be that way. Whether you're starting the Fat Flush diet and fitness plans at age twenty, forty, sixty, or even older, you can rest assured that this way of eating and working out will generate enormous new reserves of energy and help you to feel flexible, strong, and calm. It's certain that you will get older with every passing day—but it's far from a foregone conclusion that your body has to "wear out" or "give in." Remind yourself that taking care of your body in this way will enable you to come through for yourself—*and* for your partner, children, and grandchildren!

Stop exercising immediately and consult your doctor if you experience any of the following symptoms:

- Severe shortness of breath with light to moderate activity

- Muscle cramps

- Coughing or wheezing

- Chest pain, chest tightness, or pain radiating down your arm

- Irregular, rapid, or fluttery heartbeat

- Dizziness

- Excessive perspiration

- Sharp pain

- Problems walking after exercise or a fall

- Nausea

- Extreme fatigue

- Numbness

Stimulating the Lymphatic System Is the Key to Effective Exercise and Weight Loss

If the liver is the body's filter, the lymphatic channels are its drainage system. Most of us are familiar with the cardiovascular system and its role in our well-being, but the lymphatic system needs to get a better press agent! Despite the crucial importance of this system to our health—and notwithstanding its central role in weight gain—many of us have barely heard of it.

Improving the health of the lymphatic system is the cornerstone of the Fat Flush Fitness Plan, so we'll be returning to this concept again and again throughout this book. For now, let's start with the basics.

The bloodstream carries oxygen and nutrients to every cell in the body, bathing them in a rich fluid that is pumped through the body by the heart. Then, a watery fluid carries away waste products and toxins from the cells, about 85 percent of which returns to the bloodstream. The remaining 15 percent flows into the lymph system, where it eventually reaches the heart.

The word *lymph* comes from the Latin word for "water goddess," in honor of the fluid's watery nature. Healthy lymph is transparent, with a slight yellow tinge and a vaguely opalescent sheen. Unlike blood, which is pumped by the heart, lymphatic fluid has no pump. Instead, what moves the lymph through its many ducts and channels is exercise.

That's right, exercise. The behavior of the lymphatic system is one of the ways we know that nature intended us to be active, vigorously moving creatures, not sedentary couch potatoes or frantic workers chained to our desks. Mother Nature was so sure we'd be constantly moving—gathering food, building shelters, running away from wild animals—that she seems to have assumed that the lymph system could rely on voluntary activity, rather than on the involuntary constant beating of a heartlike pump. She didn't count on eighty-hour work weeks and twenty-four-hour cable television.

Ideally, our lymph moves through a complex network of needle-thin tubes known as lymphatics, collecting excess fluid from cells all over the body. Different body parts produce different types of lymph: protein-rich

---

Valid Exercise Excusers
When your immune system is working overtime to fight an infection, exercise adds to its burden. So don't exercise when:

- You have a fever. You're better off taking a break than breaking a sweat. When your body temperature rises above 99 degrees Fahrenheit, your risk of heart failure or dehydration during exercise vastly increases. So wait until your temperature has been normal for at least twenty-four hours before you start to exercise again.

- You're taking antibiotics. A study reported in the *American Journal of Sports Medicine* found that at least one antibiotic, ciprofloxacin, can damage tendon tissue, increasing your risk of injury when exercising.[2] Other antibiotics may cause additional problems. If your doctor has prescribed a long-term course of antibiotics, be sure to ask him or her about possible side effects with exercise and find out when it's safe to start or resume your exercise routine.

- You have an intense headache. Headaches are caused by excess flow of blood to the vessels in the scalp and neck. So even if all you've got is a migraine or tension headache, exercise is going to make you feel worse.

- You have cold or flu symptoms, especially coughing, achiness, and fatigue, or you have a severe sore throat, bronchitis, or pneumonia. Exercise invites your lungs to work extrahard, expanding your lung capacity and flooding your body with healing oxygen. But if you've got a cold, flu, or related disorder, all that deep breathing will set off a round of coughing that will only make you feel worse. And when you have an infection—in your lungs, your throat, or anywhere else—your body needs all its resources to fight off the illness. So heed the message your body is sending you and give yourself the rest you obviously need. You'll exercise all the better when your infection is defeated.

When you do resume your routine, start slowly at about half your normal rate before the illness. And stop as soon as you get tired. Overdoing it is only going to put you back in your sickbed!

---

fluid from the limbs; lymph full of white blood cells from the bone marrow, thymus, and spleen; and, most important for our purposes, high-fat lymph from our intestines. Fat is the only food element that moves through the lymphatic system. The proteins and carbohydrates that we ingest go right from the intestines into the bloodstream, but the intestinal lymphatics draw fat into the lymphatic system before it reaches the blood.

Now, what happens when the lymph isn't flowing properly? First, the excess fluid that isn't draining from our tissues causes them to swell. As Ann Louise explained in *The Fat Flush Plan*, these bloated, water-logged tissues can add up to 10 or 15 pounds to your weight, and cause you to swell two extra dress sizes.[3]

Also, poor lymphatic circulation means that the nutrients we ingest don't get properly absorbed. Picture a single body cell as it is bathed in nourishing fluid from your bloodstream. This little cell is fed by the water, proteins, and other molecules that leak from the capillaries—tiny arteries that drain into body tissues. But if the tissues are already full of liquid, they can't efficiently absorb those nutrients. It's like having a backed-up drain—no more water can get into the sink because it's already full. The function of the lymphatic system is to continually drain excess liquid, so that new blood, with its new nutrients, has room to flow into the cells.

Obviously, if the new blood has trouble reaching your cells, you won't absorb its nutrients very efficiently, and so you'll need to eat more to obtain the same nutritional benefits. In fact, you might be relatively malnourished, despite the high-quality food you are consuming. That's why the Fat Flush fitness program is so helpful for both losing weight and gaining energy. By assisting the lymphatic system to drain fluids more effectively, it enables each cell in your body to absorb available nutrients, making the best use possible of every calorie you consume.

As you visualize this system, you'll begin to understand why doctors recommend these steps to achieve good lymphatic health:

1. Drink lots of high-quality liquids. Both your blood and your lymph need water to help keep the fluids flowing. Without a "high water table" to keep things moving, your body tissues can't drain properly and become swollen with fluids. Ironically, drinking more water actually means you'll retain less. The Fat Flush Plan accomplishes this goal with a unique lymph-cleansing combination of pure, unsweetened cranberry juice diluted with water. (The sweet cranberry juice cocktails you may be used to won't work for this purpose!)

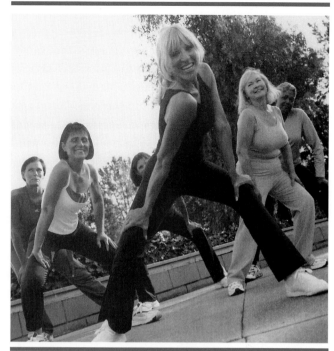

2. Eat a proper balance of lean proteins, slow-acting or low-glycemic carbs, and the right kinds of fats. Ann Louise explains in *The Fat Flush Plan* why the omega-3 and -6 fatty acids are essential.[4] But too much of the wrong fats, such as trans fat or hydrogenated fat, can clog your lymph system as well as your arteries.

3. Avoid pollutants, additives, solvents, pesticides, and other toxins. Remember, it's the liver's job to filter these poisons out of your system. Otherwise they end up in the bloodstream—and in the lymphatic system as well.

4. Keep moving. Again, the blood has a heart to keep pumping it through the arteries and veins, but the lymphatic system has only you. It is literally your own bodily movement—walking, running, and dancing with your legs; pumping and swinging and lifting your arms—that keeps the lymph flowing.

Another factor that impedes lymph circulation is poor posture. One of the major passages in the lymphatic system is called the inguinal canal; this is a very narrow channel in the groin through which lymph vessels and veins pass as they drain away the fluid from the legs. Although this canal is covered by a tough coating of ligament, it can nevertheless be compromised by outside pressure caused from such factors as tight clothing, excess weight, sitting for a long time, and poor posture.

If the lymph vessels and veins can't properly drain fluids from the legs, these fluids begin binding to fat cells, which then swell. This in turn causes still more backup of lymphatic fluids. Some experts believe it's this lymphatic backup that creates the appearance of cellulite, the dimply, spongy substance that appears on our hips and thighs.[5] Some also think that this type of fluid backup is the culprit responsible for varicose veins.

It's not just the inguinal canal whose function is compromised by poor posture. The largest channel of lymph in the body is located in the chest, near the heart. The thoracic duct conveys lymph into the blood, so that the white blood cells it carries can reach sites of infection and distress. This duct can be constricted, however, if you stand with a slumped back or drooping shoulders—as Emily realized she often did on her nursing shifts. Kate was surprised to learn that her sedentary lifestyle was interfering with her lymphatic flow, while Madison realized that her tobacco and caffeine habit was dumping excess toxins into her lymphatic system—and sabotaging her weight loss efforts.

The Fat Flush eating plan will help detoxify your lymph system as well as your liver, providing the key nutritional balance of lean proteins, slow-acting, low-glycemic carbs, omega-3 and -6 essential fatty acids, cran-water to aid in the thermogenic (nonstimulant) removal of excess fluids, and culinary herbs and spices. (Ann Louise also created a Fat Flush Kit of three dietary formulas that helps ensure proper nutrient intake during weight loss as well as adequate liver support. See Resources, Chapter 10.) This companion fitness plan is also designed to promote the health of the lymphatic system, through a variety of proper movements of the limbs, as well as massage and dry-brushing, which are known to promote a freer movement of lymph through all its channels.

We've also organized phase 3 of our plan around exercise so lymph friendly that we call it the Lymph-Fit/Compound Strength and Stretching Workout. This set of exercises is intended to improve posture (freeing the pressure on your inguinal canal), promote deep breathing (to keep lymph moving through the thoracic duct), and to give your feet a workout as well. It turns out that pointing your toes and working the soles of your feet are closely related to stimulating the flow of lymph in the lower half of the body. And guess what? Although we haven't yet amassed the hard scientific evidence to prove it, hundreds of women tell us that the Lymph-Fit/Compound Strength and Stretching Workout in addition to the Fat Flush eating plan seems to make cellulite disappear.

Stress—Including Excessive Exercise and Lack of Sleep—Is Probably the Most Insidious Weight Gain Factor Among U.S. Women Today

This point is always the biggest surprise to the women we work with. They may have heard about toxic livers, they're fascinated to learn about lymph—but when we tell them that losing weight involves getting more sleep, cutting back on excessive exercise, and generally creating more serenity and calm in their lives, they simply stare at us in disbelief.

Emily's reaction was typical. "I thought being active was a good thing," she told Joanie, shaking her head. "I thought at least being on my feet all day meant I was staying in some kind of shape."

Madison was even more vehement. "I can barely keep my weight down with what I do now," she said. "Now you're telling me I have to do *less*?"

Even Kate was taken aback. "I do fine on six hours of sleep a night," she said, "and while I don't like getting by with four, sometimes that's what I need to do my job. Adding a little exercise is one thing—but do I have to change my entire life?"

Joanie told Kate what we'd like to tell all of you, whether we're talking about the Fat Flush eating plan, the Fat Flush Fitness Plan, or anything else. Let's just take it one step at a time. The first step is learning a bit more about your body, so you know why stress, excessive exercise, and sleep deprivation make it so hard to lose weight.

The pioneer researcher in the field of stress was Dr. Hans Selye.[6] Selye saw life as a series of challenges to the body, which he called *stressors*. A stressor is any type of challenge, from a hard-to-open box of crackers to the death of a loved one, from a minor spat with your spouse to a 10-mile run. Anything that requires you to mobilize your resources is, according to Selye, a stressor.

As you can see, stress is not necessarily a bad thing in and of itself. Meeting challenges—whether physical, emotional, or a combination of the two—is part of the fun of life, and certainly part of what enables us to become physically fit, intellectually sharp, and generally good at our jobs. Being in a loving relationship, raising children, or embarking on a demanding career can be key components of building a rich, full life, and we'd be the last to suggest that you should "avoid stress" by turning your back on these worthwhile challenges.

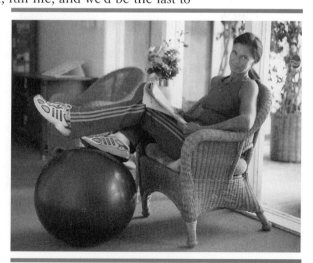

The goal is not to avoid stressors, but to understand what happens when we encounter them and then to choose the healthiest and most satisfying responses. We can choose better if we know what's going on in our bodies whenever we're confronted with a stressor, a process that Selye named the General Adaptation Response. Selye identified three phases of this response.

1) THE ALARM REACTION

Our first response to any type of stress is the famous fight-or-flight reaction, in which our bodies gear up for a short-term burst of extreme energy—ideally, enough energy to either fight an enemy or run away from it. Our adrenal glands flood our bodies with stress hormones—epinephrine (adrenaline), norepinephrine (noradrenaline), and cortisol, among others—to make our hearts beat faster, our blood pump harder, and muscles tighten up. These are precisely the reactions we need to engage in vigorous, short-term physical action in which we are literally fighting for our lives.

Note that our bodies produce these physical reactions whether we are responding to a physical danger or an emotional problem, or even a scary movie! Just imagining the feeling of stress or danger—worry, excitement, the intense anticipation of something good or bad—is enough to get our stress hormones flowing, as though our bodies were facing an actual physical threat.

Ideally, we face our challenges, respond, and then relax. The stress reaction is one of the few chemical responses in the body that doesn't have a built-in "off" switch, so we have to find a mental, emotional, or physical way to tell our adrenal glands to stop sending out stress hormones. Our biology evolved in response to physical stressors—wild beasts, hostile humans, difficult physical terrain—so the muscular effort involved in responding to these physical challenges does indeed use up the stress hormones. After this prolonged physical effort, we may be depleted and exhausted. We naturally seek sleep, proper nourishment, and a "no-stress" environment to help us restore our bodies until they are rested and ready for the next challenge.

But what about modern-day stressors—a fight with a spouse, a deadline at work, fear of not paying the bills? These stressors don't require us to engage in vigorous physical activity, so we may need to achieve relaxation through exercise—or through meditation, conscious breathing, or even a warm soak in the tub. Without some signal that the danger is over, the stress hormones remain in our bodies far longer than we need them, wreaking havoc with our metabolism and mental states.

This is problematic enough when we're talking about infrequent and short-term stressors. If, for example, you have a once-a-week production meeting at work that stresses you out, you may feel keyed up and on edge for a few hours after the meeting is over, unless you engage in aerobic activity or some form of conscious relaxation to help you "come down" from the event. Still, if that's the only intense stressor you face all week, it's probably not a big deal. But what about women such as Emily and Kate, who, like most of us, are under long-term or prolonged stress, stress that either doesn't go away or that returns repeatedly? That's when problems start, because when we're under continuous or frequent stress that isn't released through exercise, meditation, or conscious relaxation, our cortisol levels tend to stay high.

Now, high levels of cortisol are great on a temporary basis, when you want to gear yourself up for a challenge. But you don't want them in your body for long periods of time. That's because cortisol's job is to boost our energy levels, by any means necessary. If cortisol levels stay high for too long, the cortisol starts breaking down the cells in our nerves, muscles, and bones and converting them to energy. In the short term, it's a rush—in the long-term, it's debilitating.

Cortisol has another job: storing energy where the body can get at it quickly. And guess where that energy is stored? In the most accessible place, biologically—as fat. If you were facing a prolonged physical challenge—migrating across the desert, say, or enduring a long, cold winter in an Arctic village—high levels of cortisol and a continual replenishing of your body fat might make the difference between life and death. But for most of us, ongoing high levels of cortisol lead only to weight gain, fatigue, nervousness, and possibly osteoporosis (loss of bone mass).[7]

If the stress continues long enough without a break, your body may even convert progesterone into cortisol. Progesterone is a hormone that's crucial for women's reproductive health. It's involved in fertility, sex drive, and healthy passage through the menstrual cycle; it also affects our moods and our sense of balance. A shortage of progesterone may lead to osteoporosis. Still, under stress the body will readily give up progesterone if it means having more cortisol. It's as though it is saying, "How can I worry about my sex life, my nerves, and my bones, when my immediate survival is being threatened? Give me that short-term energy boost of cortisol; I'll worry about my long-term health later, when I'm safe."

To really understand the nature of cortisol, it helps to picture your prehistoric ancestors, for whom your hormonal system was really designed. These were nomadic people, living by what they could gather. Occasionally, they hunted in large groups for big game—a mammoth or another large beast that they drove over a cliff or brought down through some other group activity. Animal fat in their diets was a rare and special treat, physical stressors on their system were intense and unremitting, and the most important element of survival was adequate body fat to survive the prolonged exposure to cold, the frequent food shortages, and the low-level but continuous physical activity involved in gathering food and finding shelter.

So our bodies were designed with one basic equation in mind: body fat equals survival. And for women, body fat meant group survival as well, through the ability to bear and nurse children. Those of us with female bodies live out that legacy today, in which the default response to any stressor is the retention of body fat—and, as a result of evolution, ideally, the retention of tummy fat. In *The Fat Flush Plan*, Ann Louise explains that:

> *Cortisol activates enzymes to store fat when it contacts fat cells—any fat cells. Central fat cells are deep abdominal visceral cells, which are a quick energy source in times of stress. These central fat cells also happen to contain four times more cortisol receptors than the fat cells found right beneath the skin. Consequently, cortisol is drawn to the central fat cells, which ultimately ups fat storage in that area. Thus, every time you're stressed, you're encouraging your body to have enough reserves of fat to handle the problem.*[8]

This quick burst of cortisol—with its fat-promoting properties—occurs in response to every stressor. But what happens when you're exposed—like Emily, Kate, and most of the rest of us—to ongoing or repeated stress? If you haven't figured out a coping and relaxation strategy that works for you, you're liable to proceed to what Selye identified as the second phase of the General Adaptation Response.

2) RESISTANCE

If a stressor continues for too long, or if it recurs frequently, our adrenals start to get tired and our stress hormone levels begin to fall. If too much cortisol isn't good for us, too little is far worse. Thus, both people with high cortisol levels and those whose cortisol levels are falling are prone to a host of symptoms, including cravings for sweets, weight gain, allergies, heart palpitations, insomnia and other sleep disorders, depression, fatigue, memory problems, inability to concentrate, "foggy thinking," headaches, and nervousness. Problems before and during menstruation and menopause can also be triggered by these stages.

Suppose the stressors continue. Then, Selye believed, you move on to the third phase of the General Adaptation Response—the one that, frankly, most of the women we meet are in.

3) EXHAUSTION

By now, the adrenal glands have been pumping out stress hormones for far too long, and they're *really* tired. If they don't get some rest, their ability to produce stress hormones will be seriously compromised, putting us at risk for depression, inflammation, a compromised immune system, fibromyalgia (generalized pain), and other disorders.

Remember, when we talk about long-term stress, we mean any kind of challenge: physical, emotional, or spiritual. Financial difficulties, emotional challenges, and major life changes—even welcome ones, like falling in love, having a long-awaited child, or starting a great new job—are all possible sources of ongoing stress. So are such physical conditions as food sensitivities, parasites, glandular problems, lack of sleep, irregular sleep patterns, tissue damage, pain, and the kind of blood sugar fluctuations that can be caused by consuming refined sugar, white flour, and other simple carbohydrates. You can read more about the relationship between diet and blood sugar fluctuations in *The Fat Flush Plan*.

Guess what else can cause long-term stress? Excessive exercise. If too little exercise is bad for our cortisol levels, too much exercise may actually be worse. Although in truth, most people don't get enough exercise, some people do overtrain, creating prolonged fatigue, the sense of needing to drag through the workout, problems with concentration, sleep difficulties, and depression. Excessive exercise can also lead to elevated heart rate, greater incidence of injury, chronic muscle soreness, and an increased number of minor infections—all signs of a weakened immune system and a body that doesn't have time to repair itself. And people who overexercise often find themselves craving high-sugar and high-carbohydrate foods—which makes it difficult to lose that extra 10 pounds despite their continual activity.

When we explained to Madison the relationship among cortisol, weight retention, and female hormones, Madison nodded with sudden understanding. "That's why I had so much trouble with regular periods while I was dancing," she said. "All that exercise was messing up my hormones."

Madison was also fascinated to discover that smoking and caffeine were raising her cortisol levels (in addition to stressing her liver and lymph system), which of course makes sense if you think about the kind of energy rush that you get from a cigarette or a quick cup of coffee. (In *The Fat Flush Plan*, Ann Louise highlights the effects of nicotine, caffeine, and insufficient sleep on cortisol levels,[9] which helped Kate, too, understand why her four- and six-hour nights were hurting her health in more ways than one.)

Mindful of the many factors that can trigger cortisol, the Fat Flush eating plan contains numerous suggestions that will help balance your blood sugar levels and control your production of stress hormones. The Fat Flush Fitness Plan extends this support by preventing you from overexercising. First, you're

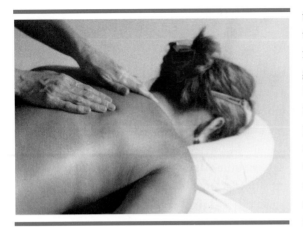

told to rest and relax during phase 1, the first two weeks of the plan, as you take a break from your regular exercise and move very gradually into mild aerobic activity. In addition, you're instructed to take weekends off throughout the entire three months of the plan. Of course, we hope you'll do something mildly active on your Saturdays and Sundays—taking a hike or a swim, going out dancing, treating yourself to a bike ride or an afternoon of in-line skating. But if you'd like to read, go to a movie, or relax at the beach, the plan makes room for you to do so.

Finally, throughout the plan, you're advised to take long, luxurious baths scented with essential oils. We hope this requirement will seem like a glorious reward to most of you—but it's not just a psychological treat. There are strong biological reasons why relaxation and aromatherapy can help bring down your cortisol levels—which will, in turn, help you lose weight.

The Fat Flush Fitness Plan: Our Invitation to You

Now that we've explored the basic biology behind the Fat Flush approach to diet and exercise, let's focus on each unique element of the Fat Flush Fitness Plan. This exercise regimen has been specially designed to support the Fat Flush eating plan, with three separate phases that correspond to the diet that is presented in *The Fat Flush Plan*.

When Ann Louise wrote *The Fat Flush Plan*, she included a basic fitness plan. This book is an expansion of that initial effort. No matter what your relationship to the Fat Flush eating plan or any other low-carb diet, this fitness approach will benefit you. We hope you'll follow the eating plan—but even if you don't, you can still derive numerous health benefits from this fitness plan. And if you're not currently on the eating plan, we invite you to consider it—now or in the future. In our opinion, the combination of the Fat Flush eating plan and the Fat Flush Fitness Plan is simply unbeatable.

The Fat Flush Fitness Plan: An Overview

Phase 1: TWO WEEKS

- Sun Salutation—five minutes, five days a week

- Mild aerobic exercise in the form of rebounding or a brisk walk, followed by cool-down stretches—twenty-five minutes, five days a week

- Lymphatic massage—half an hour, once a week

- Aromatherapy bath—twenty minutes, three times a week

Phase 2: SIX WEEKS

- Sun Salutation—five minutes, five days a week

- Rebounding or a brisk walk followed by cool-down stretches—thirty-five minutes, five days a week

- Strength ball workout, followed by cool-down stretches—twenty-five minutes, twice a week

- Dry-brush massage—five minutes, twice a week

- Aromatherapy bath—twenty minutes, three times a week

Phase 3: FOUR WEEKS . . . AND THE REST OF YOUR LIFE

- Sun Salutation—five minutes, five days a week

- Rebounding or a brisk walk followed by cool-down stretches—forty-five minutes, five days a week

- Lymph-Fit/Compound Strength and Stretching—twenty minutes, twice a week

- Lymphatic massage—half an hour, once a week

- Dry-brush massage—five minutes, twice a week

- Aromatherapy bath—twenty minutes, three times a week

All Phases of the Plan: Twelve Weeks

It's often hard to make changes in your exercise and eating habits. But think of it this way: Your current lifestyle is probably geared to making you gain or retain weight, even as you feel enervated and stressed out. The Fat Flush Fitness Plan, on the other hand, will offer you both immediate results and long-term benefits. As you cleanse your lymphatic system, detox your liver, and build up lean muscle mass, you'll discover an almost-instant boost in your energy reserves, even as you find yourself feeling calmer, more focused, and more optimistic about your life.

Meanwhile, you'll be losing weight, ridding yourself of unwanted tummy fat, losing inches at your hips, waist, and thighs, tightening up the flesh and skin along your upper arms, lifting your rear and firming up your buttocks, making your entire body more limber and flexible, and significantly reducing the appearance of cellulite. You'll discover that your body is toned, glowing, and full of energy.

Every aspect of the Fat Flush Plan is designed to boost your overall health as well as to help you lose weight and become more fit. This is a new approach to honoring, respecting, and nurturing your body. Throughout the Fat Flush Fitness Plan, you'll be eating healthy, well-balanced meals and getting eight hours of deep, restful sleep each night. You'll also keep a journal recording your activities and experiences, along with your daily food choices and eating habits. We've found that keeping a journal is an integral part of both the Fat Flush eating plan and its companion fitness plan. Journaling helps you keep track of how well you're following the plans and what the results are. Perhaps more importantly, keeping a journal helps you become more aware of your body, your eating habits, and your emotional responses to food and exercise. As you develop a closer relationship with your physical self, you'll find yourself instinctively making the diet and exercise choices that are right for you.

This entire plan can be summed up in four words: the power of now. Because honestly, now is all we have. Why should you live even one more day feeling stressed out, exhausted, and overweight? Why should you finish out the month looking less than your best? Combined with the Fat Flush eating plan, this fitness plan can help you lose noticeable amounts of weight in just the first two weeks—and the weight loss, toning, and energy boosting will continue throughout the program and for the rest of your life. So what are you waiting for? Let's get started.

The Fat Flush Fitness Plan

Phase 1: TWO WEEKS

This corresponds to "Phase 1: The Two-Week Fat Flush," a portion of the diet that focuses on supporting the liver and releasing the toxins accumulated there, in the lymphatic system, and in your stores of fat. Most women lose weight extremely quickly during this phase, which provides instant gratification and makes it easy to continue with the plan. However, this is also a time when many women feel unusually tired, as they give up the caffeine, sugar, and white-flour foods that have been providing them with "quick fixes" of temporary energy. Some women experience headaches, nausea, and other types of discomfort as they withdraw from their reliance on coffee and "high–blood sugar" foods, or as their bodies respond to the toxins that are being released from their systems. But this lasts only for a short period of time—then you'll feel downright euphoric.

This portion of the diet is also lower in carbohydrates, as we help you readjust your eating habits and recalibrate your blood sugar levels. As a result, you won't have the high-carb intake necessary for vigorous physical exercise and weight training. But your body will quickly readjust and your energy levels will skyrocket.

So phase 1 of the Fat Flush Fitness Plan can be summed up in three words: *take it easy*. If you're used to high levels of exercise, give yourself a break. If you're just getting started with a fitness routine, go slow. We'll give you more details about this phase of the plan in Chapter 3. For now, just be aware that this first two weeks is a time of transition—and, like all transitions, it requires you to be more than usually gentle and loving with yourself.

SPECIAL FEATURES OF PHASE 1:

- Mild aerobic exercise in the form of rebounding or a brisk walk, followed by cool-down stretches—twenty-five minutes, five days a week

This is your basic cardiovascular workout, the aerobic exercise that lowers your blood pressure, reduces "bad" cholesterol, elevates "good" cholesterol, and stimulates the flow of lymph. We just can't say enough good things about the many health benefits of doing this type of exercise—so we'll turn the podium over to JoAnn Manson, M.D., who studied more than 73,000 postmenopausual women at Brigham and Women's Hospital, and who has analyzed the Nurses' Health Study, an observational study of 121,000 women who are surveyed about diet, activity, smoking, and medical history.

From her work with both studies, Manson has concluded that moderate to vigorous activity for three to four hours a week lowers the risk of coronary heart disease, stroke, Type 2 diabetes, and breast cancer.[10][11] "I'm convinced from the research that a sedentary lifestyle kills you, and moderate activity like walking can be a lifesaver," says Manson.[12]

Moreover, Diane Feskanich, an assistant professor at Harvard Medical School and Brigham and Women's Hospital in Boston, found that middle-aged and older women can significantly decrease their risk of hip fractures through regular exercise. The study, published in the *Journal of the American Medical Association*, was based on questionnaires completed by 61,000 postmenopausal women aged forty to seventy-seven.[13] "Doing anything is better than doing nothing; doing more is better than less," Feskanich has said.[14]

Although you can certainly fulfill this portion of the Fat Flush Fitness Plan by walking, we urge you to consider an alternative that studies have shown to be even more effective, pleasurable, and user friendly: rebounding. We've come to call rebounding the "excuse-proof exercise" because you can do it in your backyard, your office, or your bedroom, and you can combine it with watching television, listening to music, or even talking on the phone.

You will find more on the extraordinary benefits of rebounding in Chapter 3. Meanwhile, we'll leave you with the assessment of Gerald M. Lemole, M.D., a cardiologist and author of *The Healing Diet*, a book on lymphatic health. A huge fan of rebounding, Dr. Lemole calls it "a form of exercise particularly suited to the lymphatic system."[15]

- Lymphatic massage—half an hour, once a week

The vigorous walking and bouncing you'll be doing in your cardio workout is designed to get your lymph flowing, and if you're like most of the women we work with, you'll notice the improvements right away: more energy, a loss of bloat and water weight, and—Joanie's personal favorite—clear, glowing skin. However, your poor lymphatic system has been neglected for so long, we want to give it some extra attention, so we've built in this once-a-week lymphatic massage. You can do it yourself or find someone to do it for you. You'll find detailed instructions on this technique in Chapter 7. And this is one part of the plan that you can't overdo, so if you like massage as much as most people do, feel free to build in even more sessions.

Phase 2: SIX WEEKS

Phase 2 is where we add strength training, which helps to build lean muscle mass. Increasing the proportion of muscle in your body is also an invaluable weight loss tool, because muscle is your most metabolically active tissue. In fact, lean muscle tissue metabolizes calories even when it's at rest. So if your lean muscle mass is high enough, you can be burning calories even while you're sleeping, watching TV, or relaxing in a nice, hot bath. A person with insufficient muscle doesn't receive those calorie-burning benefits—and consequently finds it harder to lose weight.

This metabolic property of lean muscle mass helps explain why a combination of diet plus exercise is the most efficient and healthiest way to lose weight. When you diet without exercising, you lose up to 25 percent of the weight as muscle or other tissue. But every ounce of muscle tissue that you lose sabotages your ultimate weight loss goal, because you're lowering your muscle-to-fat ratio—unless, at the same time you are dieting, you're building up lean muscle mass through strength training or some other means.

This explains, too, why you may find that you're gaining weight even though you're eating exactly the same way you always have. If you haven't been exercising over the years, you'll naturally have less lean muscle mass than you did in the past. The diet that was appropriate to your previous ratio of muscle to fat is no longer suitable for your current body. The good news is that you can reverse this trend by increasing your body's percentage of lean muscle.

SPECIAL FEATURES OF PHASE 2:

- Strength ball workout, followed by cool-down stretches—twenty-five minutes, twice a week

This portion of the Fat Flush Fitness Plan focuses on building up lean muscle mass using a strength ball, a 6- to 12-pound ball that's about two-thirds the size of a volleyball, with a rubber or polyurethane surface. You hold the ball with both hands and go through a series of exercises that helps expand your range of motion while creating a higher proportion of muscle to fat, toning your muscles, and stimulating your lymph flow.

Because you use both hands together, you avoid the problems of free weights, which can sometimes build up one side at the expense of the other. You also avoid the limitations of weight machines, which tend to focus on a restricted range of motion. Most important, the strength ball workout develops your core muscles—those deep in your chest, abdomen, and lower back—along with your upper body, back, and legs. As a result, you're reducing tummy fat, strengthening your abdomen, and improving your posture, which, as we've seen, takes pressure off the inguinal canal and helps your lymph flow freely.

• Dry-brush massage—five minutes, twice a week

We want to give your lymphatic system all the support it needs. So in phase 2, we've built in a quick dry-brush massage. Like the self-massage in phase 1, it will help you keep your lymph flowing freely.

Phase 3: FOUR WEEKS . . . AND THE REST OF YOUR LIFE

Here's the culmination of both the eating and exercise plans: what we hope will be an approach to diet and exercise you can sustain for the rest of your life. As you can see from checking out the summary that follows, phase 3 includes about an hour of activity per day, five days a week, with two rest and renewal days when you can either find some other kind of fun physical activity or just relax with a book. You'll stay with your Sun Salutation—the yoga-based stretching and body awareness exercise that helps keep you fit and flexible—along with your thrice-weekly aromatherapy baths that offer you a chance to relax and detox. The important thing about phase 3 is to include both cardio-friendly aerobic exercise and strength training to build lean muscle mass.

SPECIAL FEATURES OF PHASE 3:

• Lymph-Fit/Compound Strength and Stretching Workout—twenty minutes, twice a week

This set of exercises was specially designed by Joanie to promote the smooth and efficient flow of lymph throughout the body. Most of the exercises are done standing upright and barefoot, to help strengthen and stretch your spine and your abdominal muscles, which will improve your posture, thus taking pressure off the inguinal canal. This unique set of vigorous exercises is designed to use your own body as resistance, continuing the strength training benefits from phase 2. The Lymph-Fit/Compound Strength and Stretching Workout is an ideal form of compound exercise, both strengthening and stretching your muscles.

Working barefoot also enables you to take full advantage of the planter-fascia reflex, the reflex action of the fibrous tissue between your heel and the base of your toes. When this area is stiff, it can be very painful, but when you stimulate it, its numerous receptors help encourage lymph flow. Pointing and flexing your feet helps the lymph move along, potentially allowing you to overcome cellulite and varicose veins. Maybe years of doing barre work that emphasizes supple, flexible feet is why dancers seem to have such great legs!

The Lymph-Fit/Compound Strength and Stretching Workout also encourages regular deep breathing, another lymph-friendly activity. When you inhale, you create negative pressure in your chest cavity, drawing lymph in toward the thoracic duct. Remember, this is largest channel of lymph in your body, the last stop before lymph reaches the bloodstream. Poor posture and shallow breathing can constrict this duct—while the breathing and exercise of the Lymph-Fit/Compound Strength and Stretching Workout helps to open it up.

- Combination of Lymphatic and Dry-Brush Massages—half an hour, once a week; plus five minutes twice a week

Once again, the massages help keep your lymph flowing, and offering you two types of massage enables you to build variety into your daily routine.

Getting Started

Now that we've taken a look at the basics of the Fat Flush Fitness Plan and the reasoning behind it, you may be rarin' to go. If so, terrific! Move quickly through the next chapter, pausing only to note the cautions about times you should not exercise and the instructions for the journaling part of the plan.

On the other hand, if you're like many of the women we encounter, you may still have some lingering concerns, questions, or just plain hesitation. If you'd like some help getting motivated, know that the next chapter has been written with you in mind. We've done our best to answer the most frequently asked questions and to respond to the kinds of concerns that the women we work with have raised.

Either way, congratulations! Just by picking up this book and reading this chapter, you've taken the first step toward reshaping your body—and your life. Changing the way that you eat and starting or enhancing an exercise regimen isn't always easy, but we can promise you that this one *will* be rewarding. Just take it one day—or one chapter—at a time.

Flush Fitness Plan—will help you lose at least a little weight, no matter what else you do.

When these superathletic women start eating better and engaging in all the other supportive activities of the Fat Flush plans—the baths, the Lymph-Fit/Compound Strength and Stretching Workout, the elimination of caffeine and sweets—they discover that their athletic performance benefits and they relax. Once they've balanced their eating—adding moderate amounts of fruits, vegetables, omega-3 and omega-6 essential fats, cran-water, and protein to their diets; cutting out the refined carbohydrates, sugar, trans fats, and caffeine—they get in touch with their own natural energy. All of a sudden, they see that they can eat well, overcome their hunger, and still lose weight.

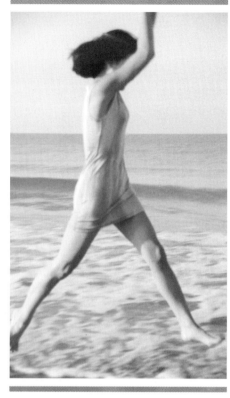

Many of these women then decide they want to go all the way, detoxifying their bodies with phase 1 of the eating plan. Because you really can't exercise vigorously during this phase—you're just not getting enough carbohydrates—you do have to cut back on your exercise for a couple of weeks. But in our experience, women who have seen how well the eating plan works are willing to give up a bit of exercise while they detox. They begin to realize that when their whole system achieves balance—the ultimate goal of the Fat Flush eating plan—they can engage in more vigorous exercise, too.

So if you're really concerned about losing your edge in a sport or competition, go ahead and jump right to phase 3 in both the diet and the exercise plans. But if you're willing to trust in our combined expertise, and to recall that each phase of the plan is carefully crafted to fit your body's needs, then take a deep breath, let go of your expectations, and start with phase 1. We guarantee you won't gain weight if you follow both the fitness and the eating plans; in fact, you'll almost certainly drop a few pounds. You won't lose any muscle in two weeks—we promise! And when you do start exercising more vigorously, you'll have increased natural energy to bring to your performance.

Remember, too, that even during phase 1, we've only regulated your activity for five days out of the week. That leaves you two free days to take that dance class or keep up with your weight training or to engage in any other type of exercise you like. Just don't overdo.

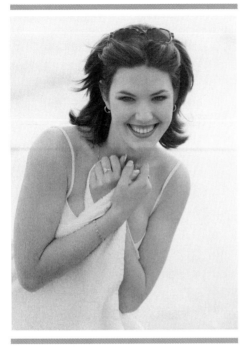

Preserving Your Skin and Muscle Tone

What about Kate's concern that losing too much weight on the Fat Flush Plan would create huge, unsightly folds of skin?

If, like Kate, you weigh less than 200 pounds, you shouldn't have anything to worry about. In fact, your skin will improve on the Fat Flush Fitness Plan, and you'll notice a tighter, firmer look to your face, neck, arms, and legs, not to mention improving the appearance of cellulite, dimpling, and rippling on your hips and thighs. Remember, you're not engaging in a starvation diet, in which your muscles are being allowed to atrophy. You're detoxifying your body, staying hydrated, feeding your vital organs—including your skin—and building up lean muscle mass, even as you flush the fat out of your system. Even if you've been overweight all your life, even if you start the Fat Flush plans over the age of fifty, sixty, or seventy, losing weight on this plan shouldn't cause sagging folds of skin if you're within 100 pounds of your ideal weight. Ann Louise has seen this time and time again on her travels across the country with Fat Flushers, both men and women, who have lost large amounts of weight.

Of course, there are always exceptions. Smoking, exposure to sun, yo-yo dieting, and just plain genetics all contribute to the development of loose skin. However, for most women on the Fat Flush plans, this is not a concern.

If you have more than 100 pounds to lose, and you're under the age of thirty-five, you still probably won't have a problem. At that age, your skin retains much of its elasticity, and you're likely to find that as you lose weight and become more fit, your skin tightens up accordingly. Again, however, sun, nicotine, previous weight gain and loss, and genetics may affect your skin tone.

If you're more than 100 pounds overweight and you're also older than thirty-five, then you may have to see how things go. Even under those circumstances, a lot of the people we've worked with have found that because the diet is so healthy and their skin benefits so greatly, they still don't have any difficulty. But it is true that if you lose vast amounts of weight over the age of thirty-five, your skin may have lost some elasticity and won't bounce back the way you'd like it to do. In that case, our advice remains the same: take it slow. By the time you've lost 60 to 80 pounds, you'll have a better idea of how your skin is responding.

Even if that's your choice, however, remember that your general appearance will already have improved in numerous ways. Joanie has noticed how virtually every woman who enrolls in her fit camps comes back with new compliments about her skin. Ann Louise has found that the same is true with women who have had only a few days of detox on the Fat Flush eating plan. This form of diet and exercise is so good for your skin, your muscles, and your overall tone, you're giving your appearance every advantage.

Keep Listening to Your Body

Many weight loss plans focus on externals—how you look, how you're shaped, into what dress size you can fit. We're all for looking good—and we promise you lots of compliments when you start the Fat Flush plans! But we believe that looking good starts with feeling good—and feeling good starts with being in touch with your body. On the Fat Flush Fitness Plan, we want you to know your body from the inside out, because in the end, that's where the real motivation for exercise comes—from within. So take fifteen minutes to move through this body awareness exercise and listen to your body. You might be surprised at what it's trying to tell you!

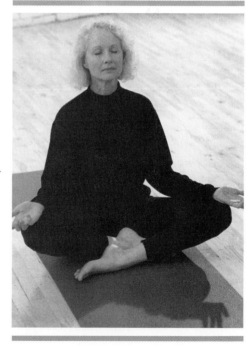

1. Find a quiet, peaceful place where you can sit undisturbed for up to fifteen minutes. Unplug the phone, turn off the radio, and insofar as possible, create a space where you can actually hear the sound of your own breath. You can sit on a chair, the floor, or even on your bed, but don't lie down—it's too easy to fall asleep. You want to be relaxed but alert, so that you can truly listen to your body. Before you begin the exercise, put a pen and paper nearby for easy access when you get to step 10.

2. Close your eyes and allow yourself to breathe deeply. Don't force your breath. Instead, think of your breath as gently floating into your lungs and then, just as gently, floating out. Slow your breathing until each inhale and exhale is eight counts long.

3. Now, listen to your body. As your lungs expand and contract, see if you can feel your heart beating. Tune into the rhythm of your heartbeat. See

if you can feel the blood pumping through your veins. Now that you know about the lymphatic system, visualize the lymph channels flowing through your body and tune in to their condition. Do you imagine them as clogged and sluggish, or as clear and flowing? Become aware of your spine. Is it a straight, powerful channel of energy, or do you feel blockages and knots?

4. Move your awareness up to the crown of your head. Notice any tension or stiffness as you move slowly down through your scalp, your face, your neck, and your shoulders.

5. Check in with your arms, your elbows, your wrists, and your fingers. Are your arms as strong and supple as you would like them to be? Do they have the full range of motion that you'd like, or are they stiff and hard to lift?

6. Move down through your chest, from your upper back through your lower back. Is your back smooth and flexible, or does it often feel stiff and achy? Can you trust your back, or do you worry about it going out?

7. Continue down through your hips and pelvis. Do you feel strong and flexible in this area? When you think about dancing, running, or making love, can you rely on your pelvis and hips, or do you have twinges, aches, pains, and stiffness in this region?

8. Move on to your thighs, knees, shins, ankles, and feet. Are your legs as powerful and vigorous as you would like them to be? Do your knees and ankles allow you to bend and stretch throughout the day? Can you walk or run as far and as fast as you would like, or are you plagued with sore shins and aching feet?

9. Bring your whole body into your awareness, from the inside out. Feel your entire physical self, and take note again of where you would like to improve strength, suppleness, and vigor. Sit for a moment with your eyes closed, soaking up this physical experience.

10. Now, open your eyes. Pick up the pen and paper, and without stopping to think about it, write down your impressions, discoveries, thoughts, and feelings. What have you learned about yourself and your body? How does this new knowledge relate to your exercise goals and plans?

Your Fat Flush Fitness Plan Questionnaire

Here's a questionnaire that can help focus some of the thoughts and feelings you accessed in the body awareness exercise. Answering these questions will also help you get in touch with your personal goals and your reasons for exercising.

1. I *do/do not* exercise as much as I would like. The main reasons
    I *do/do not* exercise as much as I would like are:

    a) _____

    _____

    b) _____

    _____

    c) _____

    _____

2. I would be happier with my relationship to exercise if

    _____

    _____

3. Three good results that can come to me from exercising are

    a) _____

    _____

    b) _____

    _____

    c) _____

    _____

4. When I finish phase 1 of the Fat Flush fitness and eating plans, I
    imagine that my body will be

    _____

    _____

5. When I finish phase 2 of the Fat Flush fitness and eating plans, I
    imagine that my body will be

    _____

    _____

6. When I finish phase 3 of the Fat Flush fitness and eating plans, I imagine that my body will be

_____

_____

7. When I think of my body in three months, I would like it to be

_____

_____

8. When I think of my body in a year, I would like it to be

_____

_____

9. When I think of my body in ten years, I would like it to be

_____

_____

10. Tomorrow, I will help myself follow the Fat Flush eating and fitness plans by

_____

_____

My Personal Fitness Goals:

_____

_____

_____

_____

_____

_____

_____

_____

Keeping in Touch with Yourself

One of the cornerstones of the original Fat Flush eating plan is journaling—keeping a daily journal to record what you eat and how you feel about it. In *The Fat Flush Plan*, a study conducted by the National Weight Control Registry is cited that found that:

> keeping a diet journal proved elemental to their [dieters'] success. . . . By taking the time to write . . . down [your thoughts and feelings], you'll reduce anxiety and stay in touch with yourself. Stress researcher Ann McGee-Cooper, Ed.D., suggests that by writing through emotions, you actually may be less likely to fall prey to stress. . . . Additional recent studies support this fact, indicating that fifteen minutes of journaling each day can cut stress levels and even bolster the immune system by 76 percent.[1]

For more on journaling, see chapter 7 in *The Fat Flush Plan* or refer to *The Fat Flush Journal and Shopping Guide*. Or, just follow these tips.

Commit to never showing your journal to any other person. Many women need some time and space that is just for them—and making time for your journal might be just the boost you need to help you make time for your workout. To know that you can be totally honest with your thoughts and feelings, though, you need to know that no one but you will ever see your journal. Give yourself this little bit of private space—and then commit to being utterly truthful. Remind yourself that the things you write may not be true for any longer than the moment it takes you to write them down. Or they might be important aspects of your life, or anything in between. Just having the space to vent, fantasize, dream, or wonder is extremely useful.

Schedule time for your journal just as you schedule time for your workout, massages, and baths. If you treat your journal as an option, you may find that every other obligation is more important—your child's homework, your husband's lost briefcase, your own need to wash out some clothes for tomorrow's big meeting. Your life is full of important duties—but your responsibility to your health and well-being is also important. Just for the twelve weeks of the Fat Flush plans, commit to building in five to ten minutes a day for your journal. If you miss a day, forget about it and move on. Otherwise, you may find that each missed day ups the ante. Now you not only have to record material from today, but from yesterday as well; and if you miss two days in a row, the third day will be truly daunting! Before you know it, you've put off journaling indefinitely, because you can't imagine finding the time to catch up. Treat a "slip" away from your journal exactly the way you'd treat a missed workout day or a day of eating "forbidden" foods—just acknowledge it, forget it, and move on.

Make your journaling time as pleasant as possible. Would it make journaling more fun if you lit a scented candle while you wrote, or put on your favorite CD? Can you journal while sipping your morning cup of tea or coffee? Maybe you'd like to take five minutes to sit in a sunny spot, or to crawl back into bed. Pamper yourself while you write, so that you come to associate journaling not with one more on a list of duties, but with giving something lovely to yourself. A sample set of journal pages can be found at the end of this chapter.

Make Your Dreams Come True

Joanie has found that one of the most gratifying aspects of running her fit camps is seeing how women's lives change after they start exercising and eating according to the Fat Flush plans. First, she says, you notice how women's skin improves, benefiting from their detoxed livers, their rejuvenated lymphatic systems, and their new intake of omega-3 and omega-6 fatty acids and cran-water. Then you start to see how well nourished and well rested they look, because they're getting eight hours sleep a night and eating more vegetables, protein, and omega-rich fatty acids. Women who starve themselves on liquid protein diets or who use coffee to suppress their appetites have that haggard look even when they become thin—but women on the Fat Flush plans are glowing with health and energy.

The best part comes when the women following both the eating and fitness plans have really gotten in touch with their newfound strength, endurance, and flexibility, and they start to make their dreams come true. Emily and Gwen were two women in their late forties who entered Joanie's fit camps at fifty and seventy pounds overweight. Their lifelong dream was to cycle through the English countryside, looking at the local gardens. One year after starting their exercise plans, they sent Joanie a postcard from England, enthusing about how much fun it was to ride six hours a day.

Cassie had never seen herself as a physical person. She got involved in fit camp because she was generally concerned about her health and weight. But as her energy levels improved, she found herself enrolling in a local salsa class. All of a sudden, she became a dance fanatic, hitting the salsa clubs every weekend, thrilled with this new activity. Likewise, Cassie discovered that she and her husband enjoyed ballroom dancing—and before she knew it, they were winning local amateur contests.

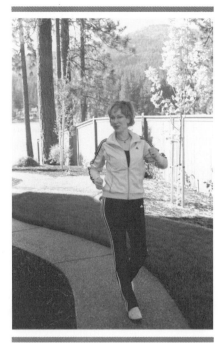

But our favorite story concerns Miriam, a woman in her early sixties with three middle-aged children. When Miriam finished fit camp, she told us that she actually had enough energy to keep up with her five- and six-year-old grandchildren. Instead of sitting on a bench watching them play in the park, she could join them in their games. "I don't know who's happier—me or the kids," Miriam said. "I do know that having this time with them is an incredible gift."

Research has shown that exercise has all sorts of mental and emotional benefits. A study published in the *Journal of Gerontology* found that women and men who exercised regularly maintained brain density longer than their sedentary counterparts, with enhanced cognitive abilities and less tendency toward depression.[2] People who exercise also report feeling more creative, flexible, calm, and empowered. Suddenly it seems possible to dream in new ways—and to make those dreams come true.

So as you embark on this new path to greater fitness and health, ask yourself what dreams you'd like to realize—and maybe even come up with some new ones. You'll find that once you start making a few little changes in your eating and fitness habits, all sorts of changes will follow in their wake. New possibilities will open up, and you'll discover a revitalized inner capacity to make those dreams come true. So go ahead, dream big. You deserve it.

Making a Promise to Yourself

All right. You've checked with your doctor, bought your new workout clothes, and told your friends and family what you intend to do. Now you're ready to get started. But if you're like the rest of us, you've probably made promises to yourself previously that you haven't kept. You may have started an exercise plan before and not stuck with it. Kate, for example, told us that over the course of her fifty-some years, she'd probably tried a new exercise plan once every three years—and she'd always dropped out three to six months later.

So what's different about this time? Well, for one thing, you're combining a fitness plan with an eating plan whose effectiveness has been proven time and time again. The stunning results that you'll get from combining the Fat Flush eating plan with the Fat Flush Fitness Plan will offer strong positive reinforcement.

This exercise plan is about making you as healthy as you can be—detoxifying your liver, cleaning out your lymphatic system, and revitalizing your skin, hair, joints, and brain. The new levels of energy, calm, and well-being that you're going to feel on this plan will also help you keep going.

Finally, this plan has lots of built-in supports—the two free days, the aromatherapy baths, and the massages. The alternating rhythm of exertion and relaxation will help sustain you, so that you come to look forward to your workout days. Rather than yet another obligation, this fitness plan makes exercise a pleasure.

The rewards are waiting for you—and we think you'll begin to notice them before even a week has passed. Still, whenever you start something new, it helps to clarify your goals and your intention. Toward this end, we suggest that you make a formal pledge to stick with the Fat Flush eating and fitness plans for the entire twelve weeks. We hope you'll want to stay on these plans for life. But start with a twelve-week commitment.

Some people like to write their pledges on the first pages of their journals, where they remain private forever. Others find it useful to get one or two friends or family members to witness their pledges, making their commitment a public affair. Do whatever works for you—but do consider writing and signing a formal pledge. You'll be surprised at how it helps you manifest your commitment to yourself.

You can write your own pledge, or use the following as a model:

I promise myself that I will faithfully follow the Fat Flush eating plan and the Fat Flush Fitness Plan for the entire twelve weeks of the plans. I will communicate to my friends, my family, and most of all, myself, that this goal is important to me. I will be forgiving of myself if I slip off the plans in any way, and I will resume the plans without beating myself up, despairing, or quitting. I will be patient with myself and others. I will ask for the support I need to follow the plans, and I will support myself by keeping a journal and staying in touch with my emotions. Most important, I will find ways to love, cherish, and support my body by getting the nutrition, rest, and exercise I need.

_____   _____

Name   **Date**

Or write it in your own words:

My Pledge

_____

_____

_____

_____

_____

_____

_____

_____

_____

_____

_____

_____

_____

_____

_____   _____

Name   **Date**

Sample Fat Flush Journal

Today's date _____

My phase _____ goal _____

_____

Measurements

    Bust/Chest _____

    Waist _____

    Hips _____

    Thighs _____

    Weight _____

Why I want to reach my goal _____

_____

_____

_____

_____

_____

_____

_____

My phase _____ goal _____

_____

_____

_____

_____

DAY 1

Date _____

Meals, beverages and snacks

Upon rising _____

Before breakfast _____

Breakfast _____

_____

_____

Midmorning snack _____

Before lunch _____

Lunch _____

_____

_____

_____

_____

Midafternoon snack _____

4 P.M. snack _____

Before dinner _____

Dinner _____

_____

_____

_____

_____

_____

Midevening _____

Supplements _____

_____

_____

Exercise _____

_____

_____

_____

_____

_____

Health and wellness notes _____

_____

_____

_____

_____

_____

Food for thought _____

_____

_____

_____

_____

_____

Sleep time _____

_____

_____

Reflections _____

_____

_____

_____

_____

_____

_____

_____

_____

_____

_____

_____

_____

Daily acknowledgment _____

_____

_____

_____

_____

_____

_____

_____

_____

_____

_____

3
Phase 1: Detox, Start Moving–and Relax!

I find the great thing in this world is not so much where we stand as what direction we are moving.

— Oliver Wendell Holmes Sr.

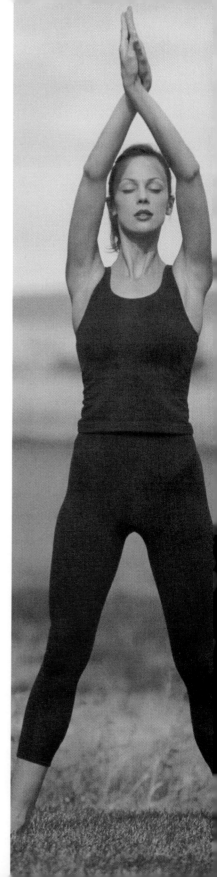

The Fat Flush Fitness Plan–Phase 1: TWO WEEKS

- Sun Salutation–five minutes, five days a week

- Mild aerobic exercise in the form of rebounding or a brisk walk, followed by cool-down stretches–twenty-five minutes, five days a week

- Lymphatic massage–half an hour, once a week

- Aromatherapy bath–twenty minutes, three times a week

Welcome to phase 1 of the Fat Flush Fitness Plan. This first phase of the fitness program has been designed to complement the Two-Week Fat Flush, phase 1 of the Fat Flush eating plan, in The Fat Flush Plan.

As you'll know from reading The Fat Flush Plan, *the first two weeks of the eating plan focus on detoxification: giving your liver a much-needed rest from caffeine, alcohol, additives, preservatives, sugar, and* the wrong kinds of fat. This initial two weeks also helps you eliminate refined carbohydrates, which—along with refined sugar and sweetened foods—trigger excess insulin production. Finally, during this initial phase you're urged to begin getting the rest and relaxation you need to reduce physical and emotional stress, and thereby lower your cortisol levels. Remember that insulin surges, excess cortisol, and a toxic, overstressed liver are all significant factors in weight gain. Correcting these imbalances almost invariably enables women to lose one to two dress sizes in the first two weeks on the Fat Flush Plan.

While virtually every woman on the plan notices increased energy levels by the end of this two weeks—and often by the end of the first few days—this transition to healthy eating can initially be tiring. You're cutting out the quick-energy fixes of caffeine, sugar, and refined carbohydrates, which can lead to such temporary withdrawal symptoms as fatigue, headaches, fogginess, and mild depression. These symptoms are usually gone within a few days, but while they last, you may experience a drop in energy.

Moreover, the very process of detoxifying can sometimes be tiring. Initially, as you flush away the toxins you've accumulated and stored in your fat, you may experience a mild reaction to these unhealthy substances. Once the toxins are gone from your body, you'll feel stronger and healthier than ever—but as they begin to depart, you may feel fatigued, mildly nauseous, and/or experience headaches.

Finally, many of us simply don't get enough sleep—and without our high-energy fixes, we suddenly get in touch with how tired we really are. We like to tell women during the detox period, "This is your real level of energy!" As you work your way through the diet and fitness plan, you'll find that your true level of energy will rise to amazing heights. Initially, however, you may feel a certain slump.

For all these reasons, we've crafted a two-week fitness phase that starts you on basic cardio-friendly aerobic activity with minimal exertion. We're not telling you not to exercise—on the contrary. Feed your body with oxygen as you do the deep *breathing and stretches of the yoga-based Sun Salutation, and the twenty-five minutes of brisk walking or rebounding plus cool-down stretches. And you've got two free weekend days when you can do anything you like, from lounging around the house with a book, to taking a hike with your family, to keeping up with your favorite dance, Pilates, or aerobics class. We just don't want you to overdo—particularly since, in this initial phase of the Fat Flush eating plan, you're getting virtually none of the carbohydrates that are essential for prolonged intense activity.*

We also want you to associate exercise with a larger vision of self-care, building in the rest and relaxation that your body needs just as much as the vigorous activity of aerobics and (in phase 2) strength training. As we explained in Chapter 1 of this book, aromatherapy baths are both relaxing and detoxifying, as they help bring the toxins in your body to the surface, where they can flow out through your skin into the water. (For more about aromatherapy baths, see Chapter 7.) Lymphatic massage—also explained in detail in Chapter 7—will also help get your lymph flowing, as will the walking or rebounding around which this phase is built.

For some of you, the activity in this phase represents a temporary decrease in the amount and intensity of your exercise. For others, even a twenty-minute brisk walk or rebounding session is more than you've been doing, and you'll have to work your way up gradually. Don't worry. Whether you're used to running five miles a day or walking only as far as the car in the driveway, we'll help you find a version of phase 1 that supports your body—and your spirit.

Sun Salutation—Five Minutes, Five Days a Week

This wonderful yoga-based warmup has so many physical, mental, and spiritual benefits that it's difficult to list them all without sounding like we're exaggerating, but we're not. The five minutes spent doing the Sun Salutation rewards you by:

- Increasing lymph flow through your lymphatic system.
- Relaxing the lymph channels (which also increases lymph flow).

- Increasing your core body temperature, which warms your muscle tissue—a good preparation for other exercise.
- Increasing your heart rate, which gets the blood flowing and improves your circulation.
- Increasing oxygen transport to all your cells.
- Increasing the circulation of fatty acids that will be used by your muscle fibers to create energy.
- Increasing the flexibility and range of motion in your muscles, tendons, ligaments, and joints.

In addition, as you become accustomed to doing the Sun Salutation, you may find yourself moving into a kind of meditative state. If you're like many people who practice this form of hatha yoga, your mind may clear, and you'll feel a sense of serenity and calm that often lasts for several hours. Meditation releases powerful hormonal messages that relax your lymphatic channels and help flush toxic fluids from your body tissues. It also seems to open up the creative and spiritual aspects of your mind.

Jeannette, a woman in her mid-forties who had never exercised before, told Joanie that after doing the Sun Salutation for two or three months, she noticed herself coming up with new ideas at work, finding solutions to problems that had been plaguing her for some time but that she had never quite been able to get a handle on. Lenore, a mother in her thirties, reported having significantly more patience with her two toddlers.

One of the great benefits of the Sun Salutation is the way in which it helps you to breathe deeply. If you feel stressed, frustrated, foggy, or simply overwhelmed, deep breathing is one of the best ways to clear your head and get back in touch with your best self.

On a physical level, deep breathing creates negative pressure in your chest cavity as you inhale, which helps draw lymph toward your thoracic duct, its last stop on its journey through your body. The thoracic duct is where waste products are removed from the lymph so they can be flushed out of your system, so you can see why deep breathing is an important aspect of detoxifying your lymph.

Deep breathing also triggers an automatic relaxation response in your body to reduce stress and cortisol (associated with food cravings and fat retention). This type of breathing also kicks up the level of oxygen in your cells, which in turn boosts your cellular metabolism—another weight loss aid. Bringing more oxygen into your body increases the level of oxygen in your brain, which clears your head and sharpens your thinking. And the activity of contracting and expanding your abdominal muscles tones and firms your midsection. Finally, when you breathe deeply and slowly, your heart rate lowers and you release muscular tension throughout your body.

One of the goals of the Fat Flush Fitness Plan is to get you breathing more deeply and slowly all the time, not just when you're doing the Sun Salutation. You'll find that both the Sun Salutation and the aerobic training will improve your daily breathing, bringing you the benefits we've just described every waking minute.

If you're curious about how deeply you're breathing at present, try this simple test:

1. Sit straight in a chair. Place one hand on your chest, and the other on your abdomen, just below your navel.
2. Inhale. Which hand moves? If it's the hand on your abdomen, congratulations! You're already breathing deeply, and the Sun Salutation will only improve what you're already doing well.

If the hand that moved was the one on your chest, don't worry. Although, like most people, you're breathing shallowly, you've got a whole world of deep breathing in store. You might consider doing one or two breathing exercises before starting to learn the Sun Salutation, so that you won't need to learn correct breathing and the physical movements at the same time. Or you can skip these exercises and go straight to the Sun Salutation on page 51. Either way, you're in for an oxygen-rich treat.

Sun Salutation: Phase 1

Although the Sun Salutation takes only five minutes, it can be surprisingly strenuous. So we've provided you with two options: the full or half salutation. If you're used to vigorous exercise, start with the full version. If you prefer to begin slowly, use your first two weeks on the Fat Flush Plan to begin with the half version. Then move on to the full exercise as you enter phase 2 of the Fat Flush Plan.

Remember, you can do this exercise at any time. Many women on our program like doing the Sun Salutation in the morning, then doing their cardio workouts later in the day. Others like to link the Sun Salutation with the cardio workout, either in the morning or the afternoon. Still others do the cardio first and save the Sun Salutation for a five-minute pick-me-up in the late afternoon or early evening. Its combination of relaxation and energizing is ideal for either starting your morning or releasing stress that accumulates throughout the day.

To Develop Deeper Breathing

If you'd like to develop deeper breathing before you start the Sun Salutation, try these simple exercises:

Option 1: T Breather Exercise

1. Sit or stand up straight, with your arms extended in front of you, palms together.

2. Inhale deeply through your nose to a count of six as you move your arms to your sides, forming a giant letter **T**.

3. Keeping your arms extended, hold your breath for a count of four.

4. Exhale through your nose to a count of six as you slowly move your arms back to the front with palms touching.

If you're not used to breathing deeply, you may find that doing this exercise makes you a bit dizzy, so start slowly at first. Repeat it just once or twice until you're sure that you can handle all that energizing oxygen that is suddenly rushing to your brain. You might want to set aside two or three minutes each morning and evening to breathe this way, maybe when you're watching TV or waiting for the coffee to brew. Once you're comfortable with this technique, move on to our complete breather exercise, which will help prepare you for the deep breathing you need to perform the Sun Salutation.

Just don't save the Sun Salutation (or any exercise) for your last two waking hours. It may energize you so much that you'll find it difficult to sleep.

A word about breathing: As you do either the full or the half version of the Sun Salutation, think of the breath as leading you, pulling you along. Your goal is to finish a movement as you finish either an inhalation or an exhalation, to hold each pose as you hold your breath, and to let the new inhalation or exhalation initiate a new movement. Ideally, it should take you about five seconds to complete an inhalation or an exhalation, and you should try to hold (where indicated) for about five seconds as well. It may take you a little while to get used to coordinating movement and breath, but once you do, you'll be amazed at how much power, energy, and flexibility comes from working with your breathing.

Option 2: Complete Breather Exercise

1. Stand up straight. Slumping forward interferes with your lymph circulation, and it makes it difficult to take a good, deep breath.

2. Identify anything that is stressing or worrying you. Then allow the disturbing thoughts to dissipate. If necessary, tell yourself, "I'll think about that as soon as I've finished this exercise."

3. Relax your arms and shoulders. Place one hand on your abdomen.

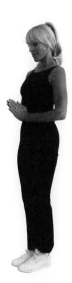

4. Slowly exhale through your nose for eight counts. Your goal is to push every last bit of air out of your lungs. But don't strain. Just let the air float out until you are completely "deflated."

5. Now, take a deep breath in through your nose, for eight counts, focusing on inflating your abdomen. Again, don't push. Think of the air floating in, just as if you were pumping up an inflatable pillow or a rubber balloon.

6. Exhale slowly through your nose for eight counts.

7. Repeat the cycle from two to ten times, allowing your attention to remain completely focused on your breathing. Most people find that after a few cycles, their breathing becomes steady and relaxed.

FULL VERSION OF SUN SALUTATION

STEP 1

Start the Sun Salutation by facing east and visualizing the rising sun. In theory, you do this exercise as the sun is just coming up, but you'll be happy to hear that we're not making that a requirement! However, it does help to visualize the rising sun, and to feel its warm, life-giving rays radiating throughout your body.

Stand up straight with your feet together. Bring your palms together, as if praying, in front of your chest. Take a moment to become aware of your entire body. Allow yourself to relax. Begin to inhale.

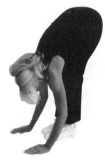

STEP 2

As you continue to inhale, extend your arms into a wide circle that starts at your sides and continues upward, until your arms are extended fully over your head. Your goal is to expand your chest fully as you press your palms together above your head. Look up at your hands, stretching your whole body upward as you hold your breath. Stay in this position for a few seconds—breath held, eyes looking upward, mind clear.

STEP 3

Exhale as you bend forward from the waist, keeping your back long and straight. Keep your palms together, and tuck your head. Your ultimate goal—though it may take you a few weeks of practice!—is to be bent completely in half.

Don't strain, though. When you've gone as far forward as you can, grab the back of your ankles, if you can reach them; or hold onto your calves, or even your thighs—however far down you've managed to get. Pull your chest gently toward your legs, keeping your chin tucked under. Hold your breath (on the exhalation) for a few seconds. Again, focus your eyes and clear your mind.

STEP 4

Inhale and move your left leg back away from your body in a wide backward step, left toes on the floor. Keep your hands and feet firmly on the ground, with your right foot (right leg is bent) between your hands. Tilt your head back and look up.

STEP 5

Exhale as you move your right leg back so it is next to your left leg (feet side by side). Straighten both legs and arms and try to keep your neck, spine, thighs, and feet in a straight line.

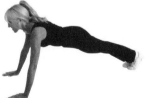

STEP 6

Hold your breath on the exhalation and slowly lower your hips to the floor until your feet, knees, hands, chest, and forehead are touching the ground. Keep your elbows bent and close to your chest.

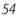

Inhale as you straighten your elbows—slowly lift your chest and stomach, keeping your hipbones on the floor. Slowly raise your head and look upward. This pose is known as the Cobra. Once your forehead is lifted, hold the position—eyes focused, mind clear.

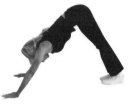

STEP 8

Exhale, keeping your arms straight, and raise your hips and align your head with your arms, forming an upward arch. You're pushing up your hips and pushing down your heels.

STEP 9

Inhale and bend your left leg at the knee, taking a long forward step and placing your left foot between your hands (as in step 4, but your left leg is forward and your right leg is back, and look up.

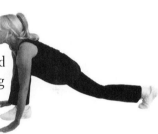

STEP 10

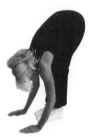

Exhale slowly, keeping your hands in place, and bring your right foot up and place it next to your left. Again grasp your legs as far as you can reach, so that you're holding the back of your ankles, calves, or thighs or you may only touch the floor in front of you at first. Bend your elbows and pull yourself in toward your legs, keeping your chin tucked under as in step 3.

STEP 11

Inhale as you straighten up. As you rise, extend your arms out to your sides and up above your head, bringing your palms together and slowly bending backward. Look at your hands and stretch upward. Hold the position—eyes focused, mind clear.

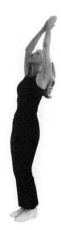

STEP 12

Exhale as you bring your arms in a circle down to your sides and then, in one slow, fluid movement, back to your chest with your palms together, so that you finish just as you began in step 1.

HALF VERSION OF SUN SALUTATION

STEP 1

Start by facing east and visualizing the rising sun. Feel its warm, life-giving rays radiating throughout your body.

Stand up straight with your feet together. Bring your palms together, as if praying, in front of your chest. Take a moment to become aware of your entire body. Allow yourself to relax. Begin to inhale.

STEP 2

As you continue to inhale, extend your arms into a wide circle that starts at your sides and continues upward, until your arms are extended fully over your head. Your goal is to expand your chest fully as you press your palms together over your head. Look up at your hands, stretching your whole body upward as you hold your breath. Stay in this position for a few seconds—breath held, eyes looking upward, mind clear.

STEP 3

Exhale as you bend forward from the waist, while keeping your back long and straight. Keep your palms together, and tuck your head. Your ultimate goal—though it may take you a few weeks of practice!—is to be bent completely in half.

Don't strain, though. When you've gone as far forward as you can, grab the back of your ankles, if you can reach them; or hold onto your calves, or even your thighs—however far down you've managed to get. Pull your chest gently toward your legs, keeping your chin tucked under. Hold your breath (on the exhalation) for a few seconds. Again, focus your eyes and clear your mind.

STEP 4

Inhale as you release your legs and lift your head away from the floor. Your body should now be in a 90-degree angle, your fingertips resting on the floor. If you can't yet manage to reach down that far, rest your hands on your shins or knees.

STEP 5

Exhale as you fold forward again, grasping the backs of your ankles, calves, or thighs.

The Fat Flush Fitness Plan

STEP 6

Inhale as you come up to a standing position, sweeping your arms out into a wide circle and bringing them up high over your head. Hold your breath as you look upward—eyes focused, mind clear.

STEP 7

Exhale as you bring your arms in a circle down to your sides and then, in one slow, fluid movement, back to your chest with your palms together, so that you finish just as you began in step 1.

Walking or Rebounding—Twenty-Five Minutes a Day, Including Cool-Down Stretches

Those of you who have already been doing aerobic exercise—walking, jogging, swimming, biking, aerobics classes, or rebounding—don't have to be sold. You already know how good it feels to give your heart a workout, to breathe deeply and break a sweat. Those of you who haven't yet done this type of exercise have something to look forward to. Take our word for it—you're in for a real treat!

In this portion of the Fat Flush Plan, you've got a choice: walking or rebounding—and we strongly encourage you to rebound. But you're not taking in many calories during this phase, so we don't want you to burn too many. If you're already swimming, doing yoga or t'ai chi, or taking regular walks, feel free to continue with those activities on your two free days a week. However, we emphatically advise against running, step classes, vigorous dance, or any other kind of intense aerobic exercise during the two weeks of phase 1 of this plan. It will both interfere with the detox process and keep you from losing weight.

Tips for Full Body Awareness During the Sun Salutation

- As you inhale, draw in the magic and joy of this moment.

- As you exhale, surrender every bit of tension.

- As you hold each pose, allow your awareness to extend to your entire body, starting from the center of your heart and radiating outward through your muscles, bones, blood, and skin.

- Feel your heart pumping and your blood moving slowly but surely through your arteries and veins.

- Visualize your lymph flowing, gleaming opal tinged with gold, as each movement pushes it along.

Remember, when you get to phase 3, you can feel free to substitute some kind of vigorous aerobic workout for one or more of the five days of walking or rebounding that we recommend here. But for the two weeks of phase 1, please stick to the walking or rebounding. We can't stress too strongly how important it is not to overdo, especially as you're undergoing the dietary shifts and detox of the Fat Flush eating plan.

How do you choose between walking and rebounding? Well, rebounding is definitely a more efficient and effective exercise, and we're going to tell you why. But once you know what your options are, it's your choice. Five days a week, you can choose either walking or rebounding. Ideally, you'll do twenty minutes of one or the other—but if you're like some of the women we've worked with, you may need a little time to reach that twenty-minute goal. If you start with only five minutes a day, don't worry. Do what you can, and add a minute or so every other day. Before you know it, you'll be hitting the twenty-minute mark like a pro.

We'd like you to do at least five minutes of rebounding on every cardio day, even if you're also walking. Feel perfectly free to focus on walking, if that works better for you, or to alternate between walking and rebounding. But if at all possible, add that five minutes of rebounding even on a walking day, because there's nothing that gets your lymphatic system moving like bouncing up and down.

Whether you choose walking or rebounding, don't forget the five minutes of cool-down stretches that follow immediately after your cardio activity. Stretching your muscles is crucial for maintaining flexibility and for preserving healthy joints. Not stretching can lead to stiffness, aches, and even injury.

Finally, whatever form of exercise you choose, take a moment to pat yourself on the back. By committing to twenty minutes of cardio plus five minutes of stretching, you are making a huge improvement in your health, well-being, and energy levels. We know it's not always easy to find the time or motivation to start a new exercise regimen—so congratulate yourself. You deserve it!

Rebounding: "The Most Efficient Form of Exercise Yet Devised by Man"

"Rebound exercise is the most efficient, effective form of exercise yet devised by man," states Albert E. Carter in his landmark book, *The Miracles of Rebound Exercise*.[1] Carter is widely regarded as the father of rebound exercise in America; indeed, he's credited with coining the term *rebound exercise*.

Did You Know . . . ?

- Excess weight has been linked to 20 percent of all cancer deaths among U.S. women and 14 percent among U.S. men, for a total of 90,000 cancer deaths per year, including cancers of the breast, uterus, kidney, esophagus, gallbladder, colon, and rectum.[2]

- In one study, the heaviest women had cancer death rates that were 6 percent higher than women of normal weight, while the heaviest men's cancer death rates were 52 percent higher than their normal-weight counterparts.[3]

- In 2000, the Centers for Disease Control found that some 65 percent of U.S. adults were above a healthy weight, while 31 percent were obese (25 percent heavier than a healthy weight).[4]

- Inactivity is one of the top four risks for heart disease, along with smoking, unhealthy cholesterol levels, and high blood pressure.[5]

- Exercise helps lower low-density lipoproteins (LDL cholesterol), which tend to stick to the sides of blood vessels and interrupt blood flow, causing heart attack or stroke.[6]

- Exercise helps raise high-density lipoproteins (HDL or "good" cholesterol), which tend to carry cholesterol away to the liver for eventual removal.[7]

- People with an active lifestyle have a 45 percent lower risk of developing coronary heart disease than people with a sedentary lifestyle, and a 35 percent lower risk of developing hypertension.[8]

- Exercise helps prevent and/or combat diabetes, joint problems, osteoporosis, gastro-intestinal problems, and cancer.[9]

- Exercise can raise the levels of such brain chemicals as endorphins, serotonin, and dopamine—neurotransmitters that help produce a sense of well-being, reduce anxiety and depression, and create a balanced sleep-wake cycle.[10]

Carter isn't the only one who advocates rebounding, though. NASA, the National Aeronautics and Space Administration, has long recognized the enormous benefits of rebounding,[11] beginning its own use of minitrampolines about twenty years ago to help astronauts recover from prolonged periods of weightlessness. NASA found that when astronauts had been in space for several months, they lost the ability to stand on their own due to degeneration of the autonomic nervous system, the portion of the nervous system that regulates such automatic activities as breathing and heartbeat. People with Chronic Fatigue Syndrome (CFS) suffer a similar decline in their autonomic nervous systems. Hence, experts such as Dr. Paul Cheney recommend rebounding to their CFS patients.

Even if you're not an astronaut, you'll find that rebounding is a remarkably effective form of exercise. It affects every cell in your body at once, and is particularly helpful to the immune system. That's because the up-and-down movement, working with the force of gravity as well as against it, stimulates lymph flow—and it's the lymphatic system that carries your white blood cells, which fight infection and help to neutralize malignant cells. Carter describes the lymphatic system as "an internal vacuum cleaner."

When you're bouncing up and down on your rebounder, your cells are participating in three separate forces: acceleration, as you rise, and deceleration and gravity, as you fall. The demands on your body's cells to adjust to each force make all your cells stronger. Your cells also experience a kind of squeezing from all the bouncing, which helps force toxins out of the cells. Meanwhile, your entire body is getting a workout, including all the vessels of your lymphatic system.

With just a few minutes a day of bouncing on the rebounder, you'll begin to see and feel results—from tighter abdominal muscles, to a higher muscle-to-fat ratio, to improved skin elasticity and tone with less visible cellulite. You'll also benefit from a stronger immune system and renewed bone mass.

Gerald M. Lemole, M.D., is a cardiologist who wrote a book on lymphatic health, *The Healing Diet*. He's a huge fan of rebounding, which he believes is particularly suited to the lymphatic system.[12] Moreover, says Dr. Lemole,

> *Exercise is a powerful conditioner of the lymphatic system. It can increase lymphatic flow threefold, thus increasing the clearance of lipoproteins, peptides, and glycoproteins from the arterial wall. . . . [B]y increasing your exercise, you can increase the circulation of HDL [the good cholesterol] in the bloodstream, thus mobilizing more cholesterol from the arterial wall.*[13]

A recent study on rebounding, conducted by researchers Colleen A. McGlone, Len Kravitz, and Jeffrey M. Janot, found that rebounding burned just about as many calories as walking on a treadmill—but without exposing people to the treadmill's danger of "impact forces," which can result in shin splints, stress fractures, and other injuries.[14] Some 80 percent of all aerobic-related injuries come from microtrauma and repetitive stresses[15]—injuries that the rebounder enables you to avoid.

Rebounding is easy to learn. The springy landing surface protects your ankles and knees, and if balance problems or disabilities keep you from bouncing upright, you can always bounce while sitting down.

Rebounding is so simple and is so much fun that you may be tempted to rebound longer than we suggest. Nevertheless, we urge you to begin slowly and progress gradually. The use of a rebounder or minitrampoline is an efficient form of exercise with virtually no harmful side effects; however, as with any new activity, you should listen to your body to avoid fatigue and discomfort. After all, you'll be on the Fat Flush Fitness Plan for the next twelve weeks— and, we hope, for the rest of your life. So for these first two weeks, especially as you're detoxing, start slowly. You've got plenty of time to up the ante!

Choosing Your Rebounder

The rebounder, sometimes called a minitrampoline, should not to be confused with the springier versions of the past. The current, more stable style enables less upward motion and more of a downward push, which in turn increases the amount of work your legs are doing. It has a firm yet giving woven mat surface, connected by coil springs to a steel frame, which is supported by four or six legs, standing about seven to nine inches off the floor.

If you want your rebounder to last a long time, check out the construction of the frame. For long-lasting durability, you're looking for a steel frame, not an aluminum one, with sturdy legs that lock securely—not ones that screw on and off. The mat should be made from state-of-the-art synthetics such as Permatron, rather than less durable canvas or nylon. Also consider:

- all-around sturdiness
- padded covering on the springs to protect your fingers
- ease of assembly
- the ability to fold up the device and put it away if space is a problem or if you want to use it while traveling

If you're concerned about keeping your balance, you can purchase a rebounder with a stabilizing bar. This is a separate attachment that extends a few feet up from the ground, which you can grab onto as you come down from each bounce. If you like, you can start rebounding with the bar in place and then later remove it as you become more confident.

There are many different brands of rebounders and minitrampolines on the market these days, with a broad range in price, but expect to pay at least $60 or more to get a good one. (To check out our top picks in today's market, see Chapter 10.) A quality rebounder should last for at least ten years.

Getting Ready for Rebounding

The goal in phase 1 is to rebound for twenty minutes a day, five days a week. As we've said so often before, we want you to begin slowly—and that goes double if you haven't been getting regular exercise before now, or if you've never rebounded before. With that in mind, we've chosen a basic move that will help you develop your balance on the rebounder device, begin to stimulate your lymph flow, and help you achieve a low-impact aerobic workout.

It takes some people a while to improve their balance while rebounding. If you're concerned about staying upright and *on* the device, put your minitrampoline near a wall that you can touch periodically, or attach the stabilizing bar.

You need to rebound immediately after doing your Sun Salutation, so your muscles will be all warmed up. Never rebound without warming up first—you could easily injure yourself.

Benefits of Rebounding

- Turns on the "internal vacuum cleaner" that is the lymphatic system, cleansing the entire body

- Fires up cellular metabolism, energizing every cell with fresh oxidants and nutrients

- Helps deliver and absorb nutrients at the cellular level

- Increases aerobic capacity and endurance

- Burns fat and calories

- Increases flexibility

- Helps improve balance and coordination

Rebounding Do's and Don'ts

DO

- Always warm up before rebounding.

- Start slowly so you can get used to the unstable surface.

- Bounce in the center of the rebounder. That way, your body weight will be evenly distributed.

- Come to a complete stop before dismounting.

- Wear comfortable, supportive clothes, such as a sports bra, T-shirt, and tights.

- Wear cross-training shoes for traction and ankle support. Socks tend to be slippery on the surface of the rebounder, and bare feet may also not grip solidly, especially as they get sweaty and damp. If you really dislike wearing shoes, experiment to see what works best for you.

- Buy a high-quality rebounder (see Chapter 10). A sturdy, well-made rebounder will last you for more than ten years and will hold up well under any type of usage.

DON'T

- Continue rebounding if you feel pain or discomfort.

- Look down at your feet while bouncing. It may cause you to lose your balance and slip.

- Attempt any gymnastic maneuvers on the rebounder. Save those for a full-size trampoline.

Warning

If you have any disabilities or ailments, including high blood pressure, a heart condition, pregnancy, asthma, or diabetes, that might interfere with vigorous activity, check with your doctor before beginning a rebounding program. If you feel any chest pain, tightness in the chest, rapid heartbeat, shortness of breath, or dizziness, stop rebounding right away; if these symptoms don't dissipate within five or ten minutes, seek medical help.

Rebounding: Phase 1

Your first two weeks are about getting familiar with the equipment and getting yourself into a regular cardio routine. This low-key beginning gives you a chance to take it slow, find your balance, and get comfortable with this exciting new form of exercise.

EXERCISE 1: WALK BOUNCE—FIVE MINUTES
1. Walk in place at an easy pace.
2. Allow your arms to hang loosely at your sides.
3. Continue for about five minutes.

EXERCISE 2: FLAT BOUNCE—FIVE MINUTES
1. Start with your feet about twelve inches apart.
2. Keeping your feet on the surface, begin a small bouncing motion. At the height of your bounce, your legs will be straight; when you land, allow your knees to bend slightly.
3. Allow your arms to hang loosely at your sides.
4. Continue for about five minutes.

EXERCISE 3: MARCH BOUNCE—FIVE MINUTES
1. Raise your left heel, keeping your toes and right foot on the surface.
2. Swing your right arm forward and left arm back.
3. Repeat with your right heel and left arm.
4. Continue marching in place for about five minutes.

EXERCISE 4: WALK BOUNCE—FIVE MINUTES
Repeat the walk bounce at a lower intensity for another five minutes, as you start to cool down. Use the last two minutes of your rebounding to gradually lower the intensity and your heart rate, so that the end of the workout serves as a preparation for the cool-down/stretching phase.

Walking: The All-Purpose Exercise

Wonderful as rebounding is, there are lots of reasons to choose walking as your phase 1 exercise—or to vary your routine between rebounding and walking. Walking is not only one of the best cardiovascular activities we know, it's also good for the lymphatic system. The combination of deep breathing and the pumping action of your arms and legs gently moves lymph fluid along, increasing lymph flow. Eventually, toxins and other debris carried by the lymph leave your body—via the skin through perspiration, via the lungs through breathing, and via the kidneys through urination.

Walking can also be done outside, as a way of getting in touch with nature, with the neighborhoods of your city or suburb, or simply getting away from home. Some women cherish their twenty-minute walks as a time to be alone and outside the home or workplace, moving freely in an environment where they have no responsibilities to anyone but themselves. It's also sometimes possible to combine walking with another agenda—walking to work, for example, or to meet a friend. If this way of building in cardio time works for you, that's terrific; just make sure to give yourself five minutes at the end of your walk to do your cool-down stretches.

What to Wear While Walking

Invest in some good walking shoes or cross-trainers—they'll give you the extra support and traction that you need on slippery surfaces, support your feet and ankles, and also serve as a key psychological marker denoting that this is your workout time.

Synthetic socks are better than all cotton—they're thin, they wick mois-

---

Did You Know . . . ?

- One-quarter of all Americans get virtually no exercise.[16]

- Even a thirty-minute brisk walk several days a week is sufficient to help women achieve "moderate" fitness levels resulting in substantial health benefits, according to an article in the *American Journal of Public Health*.[17]

- The Centers for Disease Control recommends at least two hours per week—or about thirty minutes, five days a week[18]—of walking or vigorous exercise, which reduces risk of heart disease by about 30 percent among postmenopausal women.[19]

---

ture away from your feet, and they do a great job of keeping your feet warm. Cotton socks tend to hold moisture, so that your feet stay damp and sweaty. Never layer socks if you can help it—the socks rub against one another and against your feet, causing blisters.

Synthetic clothes also wick moisture away from your body; you'll stay damp and sweaty in cotton clothing.

Basic Guidelines for Good Walking

1. Practice good posture. Walk with your chest up and your shoulders back and down so that your lungs stay open and your breathing benefits.

2. Hold your head up and focus your eyes about ten feet ahead. This will further improve your posture, which will in turn help get oxygen to your muscles and stimulate your lymph flow. You'll also reduce neck strain and excess fatigue.

3. Put your arms to work. Squeeze your shoulder blades together, bend your elbows 90 degrees, and swing your arms from the shoulder in a smooth, forward motion. Don't swing them across your body—that closes your chest, puts pressure on your heart, and interferes with breathing. Keep your left arm moving forward with your right leg, and vice versa. Your elbow should remain bent throughout. Vigorous arm movements stimulate lymph flow in the upper part of your body, just as your leg movements help pump lymph upward from your lower body.

4. Relax your knees. That reduces both stress to the joint and the potential for injury.

Monitoring Your Walking

Sometimes it can be hard to tell the difference between a casual stroll, a vigorous walk, and an overly vigorous workout. If you're concerned about whether you're maintaining the right level, choose one of these four ways to monitor your exercise intensity.

TARGET HEART RATE
Your goal is to get your heart working at 60 to 80 percent of your maximum heart rate. To find your maximum heart rate, subtract your age from 220.

Example: Age 40: 220 − 40 = 180. 180 is the maximum heart rate.
60 percent of 180 = 108—low end of training zone
80 percent of 180 = 144—high end of training zone.

You can measure your heart rate by taking your pulse at your neck or wrist. Count your heartbeats for ten seconds, starting with zero. Then multiply that figure by 6. If your heart rate is below your target zone, you need to speed up your pace. You might also want to swing your arms harder or more frequently. But if your heart rate is above the zone, slow down. You'll notice that the longer you exercise, the lower your heart rate falls; the exercise that had your heart pounding like a jackhammer during Week 1 will barely make a dent during Week 4. So give yourself some time to reach your exercise goals. Pushing yourself too hard might cause an injury or excessive fatigue that will only delay your progress in the end.

PERCEIVED EXERTION

This approach simply requires you to ask yourself how you feel as you walk. Are you breathing hard? How fast is your heart beating? Are you sweating? Are you getting tired? Rate each sensation on a scale from 1 to 10:

1–2 Very, very light exertion
3   Very light
4–5 Moderate
6–7 Somewhat hard
8   Hard
9   Very hard
10   Very, very hard

Your goal is to fall consistently in the 4 to 7 range—though you may have to increase your exercise rate to keep presenting challenges for yourself!

TALK TEST

The Talk Test is the easiest way to monitor intensity. You should be able to walk at a pace where you can speak a few sentences but would find it difficult to carry on a long conversation without becoming breathless. If you find that talking nonstop is as easy as if you were sitting down for a long chat, pick up the pace!

HEART RATE MONITORS

Heart rate monitors are easy to use, accurate, and provide a lot of information. They're probably the fastest, simplest, and most reliable way to monitor your exercise intensity (though some people prefer not to mechanize this area of their lives, relying instead on their own bodies' sense of what's enough and what's too much).

Note: *If at any point you feel undue pain, fatigue, or shortness of breath, slow down. If you experience nausea or dizziness, stop immediately.*

Walking: Phase 1

Your goal in phase 1 is to walk briskly for twenty minutes a day, five days a week. If you can't walk a mile in twenty minutes without stopping or becoming so breathless you can't talk, then start with a brisk five, ten, or fifteen minutes and work up to twenty minutes gradually. Just make sure you walk briskly for five days a week.

However you arrange your walk, use the last two minutes to gradually lower the intensity of your pace, bringing down your heart rate gradually. In that way, the end of the walk serves as an effective preparation for your cool-down stretches.

Breathe While You Walk

As we saw during the Sun Salutation, deep breathing can multiply the power of an exercise considerably, bringing innumerable physical, mental, and spiritual benefits. If you like the idea of a meditative walk, one that expands your lungs, clears your mind, and oxygenates your cells, try the following "walking-breathing" exercise to further stimulate your lymphatic flow:

Benefits of Walking

- Stimulates lymph flow and strengthens the immune system

- Increases circulation, which also boosts the health of the lymphatic system

- Moves the lymph fluid by the pumping of your arms and legs

- Diminishes unsightly cellulite

- Raises HDL, or "good cholesterol"

- Improves cardiovascular endurance

- Helps prevent bone loss and osteoporosis

- Improves mood and reduces stress and depression

Walking Do's and Don'ts

DO

- Always warm up before walking with the Sun Salutation.

- Start at your current fitness level. There's nothing to be gained by pushing yourself or pretending you're at another level—just do what you can. You'll notice signs of progress soon enough!

- Whether you've bought special exercise shoes or are simply wearing comfortable street shoes, make sure your shoes are good for walking—rubber soles, no heels, sufficient ankle support. Sore feet or a twisted ankle will make it that much harder to keep up with your workouts.

- Consult your doctor if you develop any unexplained ongoing discomfort.

- Stop walking immediately if you experience nausea, dizziness, or a sharp pain in your chest.

DON'T

- Exaggerate your stride. Your normal, comfortable length is just fine.

- Overarch your back or lean forward excessively. Standing straight makes it easier to breathe and helps strengthen the muscles in the lower and upper back.

- Overdo it after illness or inactivity. Even if you're used to a vigorous routine, take it easy when you start again—especially if you're also detoxing.

- Exercise through sharp pain. A little ache is one thing, but stop and solve the problem if you notice anything sudden or severe.

- Become dehydrated. Don't drink too much while you're walking, but do have a big glass of water before you start and have some water ready for when you're done.

1. Assume your best posture, standing upright, arms hanging loosely at your sides, chest open. Exhale deeply, to clear your lungs.
2. Start walking, right foot first, as you inhale through your nose for four forward steps.
3. Hold your breath for two forward steps.
4. Exhale through your nose for four forward steps.
5. Hold the exhalation for two forward steps.

Repeat the routine as you continue to walk, adjusting the count to your own pace if necessary. The goal is to breathe through your nose—which circulates more oxygen into your brain—and to establish a regular rhythmic breathing pattern and stimulate increased lymphatic flow.

Cool-Down Stretches

One of the most crucial parts of your workout—and one that you'll continue throughout the entire twelve weeks of the Fat Flush program—is the cool-down stretches. Stretching keeps your connective tissues elastic. It also helps your body flush out the lactic acid that accumulates in your muscles after exercise—the same lactic acid that contributes to achiness. Finally, stretching improves the range of motion in your joints and muscles and helps relieve stress and prevent injuries.

Stretching is especially important as we get older. As we age, our joints tend to lose some of their flexibility, but this tendency can be combated by regular stretching. The younger you are when you start stretching, the more flexible you'll be as you get older. If you're over age fifty and just starting to stretch, though, don't worry. It's never too late to benefit from slow, luxurious stretches!

The Fat Flush fitness stretching routine focuses on the *static stretch*—a slow, gradual, and controlled elongation that brings the muscles through the full range of motion and holds them for fifteen to thirty seconds in the furthest comfortable position (without pain). To stretch properly:

- Stretch your muscles when they're *warm*, not cold. That's why we have you do your Fat Flush fitness stretching routine right after your cardio activity when your large muscles are warm and flexible.
- Focus on the muscle you're stretching.

- Breathe deeply while you stretch. If you inhale as you begin your stretch and exhale as you hold your stretch, you'll find that your muscles extend comfortably even further. For stretches that require you to bend forward, exhale as you bend forward and inhale slowly as you hold the stretch.
- Move into the stretch until you feel a slight tension—but no pain. The stretch should feel good, even if makes your muscle feel *slightly* achy.
- Hold the stretch for ten to thirty seconds. If you are a beginner or have rarely stretched before, start with ten seconds and gradually increase to thirty seconds.
- Release the stretch slowly. Never bounce or jerk out of a stretch; that can trigger the stretch reflex, which causes the muscle to tighten, rather than relax, to protect itself from injury.

> **Benefits of Stretching**
> - Helps stimulate lymph flow
> - Increases circulation
> - Floods the body with oxygen
> - Helps reduce muscle soreness
> - Helps you relax, physically and mentally
> - Increases flexibility of joints and ligaments
> - Increases your range of motion

Although stretching may feel a bit odd if you're not used to it, you'll soon find this routine becoming second nature, so that you can focus not on the movement but on your body itself. And if you'd rather replace the routine we've outlined here with your own yoga or athletic stretches, feel free. Just make sure you're taking five minutes to stretch and cool down after each twenty-minute cardio workout.

Stretching: Phase 1

Prepare for your stretching by taking the last two minutes of your cardio workout—whether rebounding or walking—to gradually slow down. By the time you finish your aerobic activity, your breathing should be almost down to normal, as should your heart rate.

Then continue with the Fat Flush fitness stretching routine.

SHOULDER/ARM STRETCH

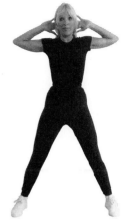

1. Place your hands on the back of your head, palms facing forward.
2. Press both arms back until you feel the stretch in your chest and shoulders.
3. Hold for ten seconds.
4. Repeat three times.

TRICEPS STRETCH

1. Raise your left arm straight up, then bend your elbow so your forearm rests against the back of your head.
2. Hold your elbow with your right hand.
3. Pull the elbow until you feel the stretch on the back of your left arm.
4. Hold for ten seconds.
5. Switch arms and repeat.
6. Stretch each arm three times.

UPPER BACK STRETCH

1. Stand with knees slightly bent, arms extended in front of your body and your hands clasped together.
2. As you reach forward with your arms, round your mid- and upper back.
3. Drop your chin to your chest and pull your hands away from your body as you resist.
3. Hold 10 seconds.
4. Repeat three times.

QUADRICEPS STRETCH

1. Stand with your left hand resting on a wall or back of a chair, left arm extended, your body perpendicular to the wall.
2. Bend your right leg behind you.
3. Grasp your right ankle with your right hand.
4. Keep your right knee pointed toward the ground and your hips pressed forward.

Stretching Do's and Don'ts

DO

- Move slowly in and out of the stretch.

- Breathe slowly, deeply, and rhythmically.

- Check with your doctor before doing any stretching if you have osteoporosis, arthritis, or other bone or joint conditions.

DON'T

- Bounce when stretching.

- Continue to stretch when you feel any pain that is greater than a mild, relatively pleasant ache.

- Hold a stretch for more than thirty seconds.

5. Pull your ankle toward your buttocks.
6. Hold for 10 seconds.
7. Switch legs and repeat.
8. Repeat three times for each leg.

CALF AND HIP STRETCH

1. Put your hands on your hips.
2. Take a big step forward with your right foot, bending your right knee and going into "lunge" position. Don't extend your knee beyond your toes.
3. Straighten your left leg and try to keep your left heel flat on the ground.
4. When you feel the stretch in your left calf, hold for ten seconds.
5. Switch legs and repeat.
6. Repeat three times for each leg.

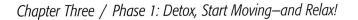

Rest and Renewal Days: Phase 1

One of the unique features of the Fat Flush Fitness Plan is the two rest and renewal days built in to the seven-day week. While you're booked for five solid days of Sun Salutation, cardio workout, and cool-down stretches, you're also given two free days to use as you choose.

Some women love to keep up with their old routines on these days, swimming, taking a dance class, or weight training. Others enjoy exploring new kinds of activity—a hike in the woods, perhaps, or a day at the beach with their children. Still other women welcome the chance to curl up with a good book or to simply sit in a park, enjoying the peace and quiet. And of course, if you're responsible for young children, your weekend may be so crammed full of trips to their soccer games or piano lessons that you welcome the chance to forget about your workout until Monday rolls around.

Whatever you choose to do on your two free days—and whether you take them together on the weekend or space them out throughout the week—we urge you to give yourself at least one satisfying treat. Whether your idea of a good time is a trip to a museum, a few hours outdoors, or a long, hot bath, build in some time for being good to yourself. Life is too short not to do so.

Meanwhile, each week of phase 1 includes three aromatherapy baths and one lymphatic massage. For more details on these features of the Fat Flush Fitness Plan, check out Chapter 7.

Finally, remember that getting enough sleep, eating well, and keeping up with your journal are crucial components of both the Fat Flush eating plan and the Fat Flush Fitness Plan. You won't lose weight if you don't— and you won't feel rested, restored, and well nourished, either.

Now, make out your workout calendar, so you know just how you'll accomplish your workout goals during the next two weeks! Some women find it helpful to post their workout calendars where their families can see them. Others prefer to keep their calendars private. Just make sure that you're building in time to nourish your body, mind, and spirit on every single one of the next fourteen days.

My Fat Flush Fitness Plan Workout Calendar: Phase 1

	Monday	Tuesday	Wednesday	Thursday	Friday	Saturday	Sunday
8 A.M.							
9 A.M.							
10 A.M.							
11 A.M.							
Noon							
1 P.M.							
2 P.M.							
3 P.M.							
4 P.M.							
5 P.M.							
6 P.M.							
7 P.M.							
8 P.M.							
9 P.M.							
10 P.M.							

My Fat Flush Fitness Plan Workout Calendar: Phase 1

	Monday	Tuesday	Wednesday	Thursday	Friday	Saturday	Sunday
8 A.M.							
9 A.M.							
10 A.M.							
11 A.M.							
Noon							
1 P.M.							
2 P.M.							
3 P.M.							
4 P.M.							
5 P.M.							
6 P.M.							
7 P.M.							
8 P.M.							
9 P.M.							
10 P.M.							

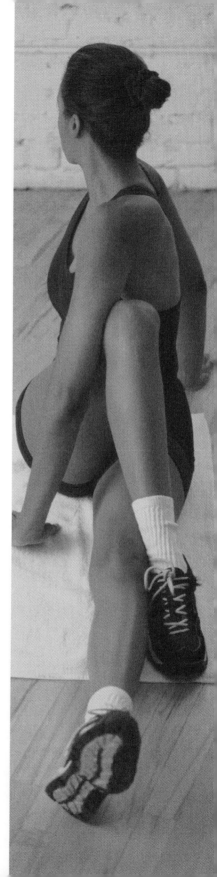

4
Phase 2: Build Lean Muscle Mass

There is only one corner of the universe you can be certain of improving, and that's your own self.

—ALDOUS HUXLEY

The Fat Flush Fitness Plan—Phase 2: SIX WEEKS

- Sun Salutation—five minutes, five days a week

- Rebounding or brisk walking, followed by cool-down stretches—thirty-five minutes, five days a week

- Strength-ball workout, followd by strength ball stretches—twenty-five minutes, twice a week

- Dry-brush massage—five minutes, twice a week

- Aromatherapy bath—twenty minutes, three times a week

Now you're entering phase 2 of the Fat Flush Fitness Plan. By now, your liver has been detoxed, your lymphatic system is cleansed, and you're starting to add back some friendly carbohydrates into your diet. You've probably noticed a huge surge of energy from the detox you've undergone in phase 1, not to mention numerous benefits from the cardio, stretching, and relaxation built into phase 1 of the Fat Flush Fitness Plan. If you're like most of the women we've worked with, you've lost from 6 to 12 inches—or maybe even more; your skin is glowing; you're more relaxed, energized, and centered; and you're ready for the next step.

Welcome to phase 2! In this portion of the Fat Flush Fitness Plan, you'll continue your Sun Salutation, your cardio plus stretches, and your aromatherapy baths. Instead of the lymphatic massages, you'll want to try some dry-brushing, which we explain in more detail in Chapter 7. You'll extend your cardio workouts another fifteen minutes or so, and you'll be adding a key component that will eventually become part of your lifelong fitness plan: strength training, to build lean muscle mass.

Because lean muscle mass is metabolically active—it burns calories even while you are at rest—one major fitness goal is to increase the proportion of lean muscle mass in your body while decreasing body fat. Of course, you need some body fat—in your breasts, your tummy, and as an allover protective coating. But you probably don't need as much fat as you're carrying, and you'll benefit from adding lean muscle mass in two ways. First, you'll find it easier to lose unwanted weight and to keep it off. Second, you'll feel your whole system sing with an energy that simply demands to be used up physically—through your workouts, on the dance floor, hiking in the woods, running around with your kids, or even taking long, thoughtful walks through your favorite museum. You will build strength and stamina in phase 2 . . . so let's get started.

Making Phase 2 Work for You

We've chosen six weeks as a ballpark figure for the length of time you should expect to stay in this phase of both the Fat Flush Fitness Plan and the Fat Flush eating plan. But if you've got more than 50 pounds to lose, you might want to stay on phase 2 of the eating plan a while longer.

It's perfectly safe to stay on phase 2 of the eating plan for up to six months, or until you've achieved your weight loss/inches loss goal, whichever comes first. However, don't stay on phase 2 of the fitness plan for more than the six weeks we've laid out in this chapter. Even if you're still eating at the phase 2 level, move on to the phase 3 workout we've described in the next chapter. Your phase 2 diet provides more than enough energy to make that work.

Strength Training: Shape Your Body and Boost Your Metabolism

When Marylou first started attending Joanie's fitness camp, she turned pale at the thought of working out with a strength ball. Joanie explained that strength balls were a useful alternative to training with free weights or machines. They also help you work through your body's full range of motion, building strong muscles, healthy connective tissue, and powerful, flexible joints.

Still, Marylou was reluctant. "Maybe I do need to lose a few pounds," she said, "but I don't want to look like a bodybuilder. What if I just upped my cardio time and left the strength ball alone?"

Joanie was quick to reassure her that the strength ball workout would not give Marylou the big, bulging muscles she feared. Instead, she'd be trim and toned. Men bulk up when they work out because of testosterone, the male hormone—but we women have only about one-tenth as much testosterone in our bodies. Not all men bulk up anyway—your body's response to weight training is largely a matter of DNA—but generally, that visible, bulky muscle mass is a male characteristic that women simply don't have to worry about. Moreover, some of the bodybuilders whose pictures you've seen— male and female—use anabolic steroids to gain muscle mass, and we certainly won't be recommending that you do that!

Meanwhile, Joanie told Marylou that if she continued to lose weight without doing some strength training, she ran the risk of breaking down muscle as well as body fat. As you learned in Chapter 1, our bodies are programmed to hold on to body fat, especially in response to activity. During most of the time that humans have been on earth, they've had to endure ongoing stresses of heat, cold, hunger, and travel, and without the easy access to fat in their diets that we have today. Body fat for both sexes was a necessity for surviving a nomadic, rigorous existence. For women, body fat was even more important: it was what enabled us to conceive, bear, and nurse children without depleting our own resources to the point of death.

As a result, our bodies are constructed to sacrifice muscle long before they let go of fat—which is why any diet or weight loss plan must include some kind of muscle-building component to replace the tissue we're losing.

Without exercise and physical activity, you'll lose 20 to 50 percent of your muscle mass over the course of your adult life.[1] We all slow down a little bit as we age, but losing huge amounts of muscle mass means a major slowdown. So if you've been feeling unusually tired and overwhelmed lately, especially if you've been trying to diet, it may simply be that the accumulated loss of muscle tissue has finally caught up with you.

Studies by Wayne Westcott, Ph.D., research director at the South Shore YMCA in Quincy, Massachusetts, confirm the role of strength training in creating muscle and reducing fat. In one study, Westcott compared the muscle gain and fat loss of two groups of participants who exercised for eight weeks. One group did only endurance (cardio) exercise, while the other did endurance (cardio) plus strength training. The endurance-only group had no change in muscle weight and only a 4-pound change in body composition (ratio of muscle to fat), while the endurance plus strength training group had a 2-pound gain in muscle weight and a 12-pound change in body composition.[2]

If a loss of muscle mass is related to aging, the release of human growth hormone (HGH) is part of what keeps us youthful. Growth hormone is secreted by our pituitary glands in different amounts throughout our lives. As the name suggests, it's most crucial during infancy, childhood, and adolescence, signaling our bodies to keep adding muscle, bone, and other tissue as we grow up. Remember as a kid when your folks told you that protein-rich foods—meat, fish, milk, and beans—would help you grow? Well, growth hormone is a crucial part of synthesizing that protein into muscle—as well as into thick hair, the collagen and elastin that gives you lovely skin tone, and the immune cells that protect you from disease.

Another key benefit of strength training is its role in building healthy bones and preventing osteoporosis. Most of us tend to forget that bones are made up of dynamic living tissue that is constantly being worn away and restored, just like the tissue in the muscles, cardiovascular system, and brain. Osteoporosis results from a loss of bone mass—the failure of the body to restore the sturdy tissue that makes up our skeletal system.

Weight training creates and maintains bone strength in two ways. First, weight-bearing exercise, in which your bones are forced to bear either the weight of your body or the additional weight of a strength ball, free weight, or machine weight, encourages your system to strengthen and develop bone. Walking is a form of weight-bearing exercise, but strength training is even more effective.

Second, researchers have discovered that when muscles contract—as during strength training—the stress of the contraction is transmitted to the neigh-

- Your metabolic rate—the rate at which you burn calories, even during sleep—will go up.

- You will have more mitochondria, those central powerhouse units in the muscle cells where fat and calories are primarily burned.

- Your lymphatic flow will be increased.

- You will gain muscle strength and endurance.

- You will lose weight and gain muscle mass.

- Your body composition will shift, with a higher proportion of muscle to fat.

- Your bones will be strong and sturdy, with far less chance of osteoporosis.

- You'll have better coordination and balance.

- You'll be less prone to fatigue.

boring bone. This stress in turn creates an electrical charge within the bone, which stimulates the activity of the bone-building cells, or osteoblasts. This response in bone is what stimulates bone formation and prevents bone loss.

We hope we've sold you on the enormous benefits of strength training! Marylou was certainly convinced—especially when Joanie pointed out that she wouldn't be on phase 2 for the rest of her life. Eventually, she would move on to phase 3 of the Fat Flush eating plan, with its greater variety of carbohydrates. "You'll need some lean muscle mass to metabolize the nutrients you're taking in," we told her. "Otherwise you'll be likely to gain back some of the weight you've worked so hard to lose."

Remember, lean muscle mass is metabolically active *even at rest*. That means your muscle mass is burning calories even while you're watching TV, sitting in the park, or getting eight hours of sleep. It's this metabolic activity that enables you to keep weight off after you've lost it. So give your body a fighting chance and make some time for strength training in your workout.

Discovering Your Unique Abilities:
Differences During Strength Training

Keisha was a tall, long-limbed young woman in her midtwenties who enrolled in Joanie's fit camp at the same time as Pat, a short, round woman of about the same age. Both Keisha and Pat had about 20 pounds to lose, and both had done some cardio work—but no strength training—before they started the camp.

To Keisha's dismay, Pat seemed to make far more progress when it came time to use the strength ball, even though both women had started out at about the same fitness level. Pat took to the strength training like a duck to water and soon had slender, firm muscles to show for all her hours working out with her 10-pound strength ball. Keisha, meanwhile, struggled even to lift a 6-pound ball. Though she insisted that she put in the same number of hours training as Pat, it seemed to take her far longer to achieve the same results.

What Pat and Keisha didn't realize was that people are simply built differently—and these differences can affect the speed and ease with which they progress through strength training. For example, we all have two different types of muscle fibers: slow twitch and fast twitch. Most of us are born with a relatively equal combination of both types, but some of us inherit more of one than the other.

Slow-twitch muscle fibers produce low levels of force for a long time. They're the muscle fibers we rely on for endurance. Most world-class marathon runners, for example, have a relatively high ratio of slow-twitch fibers.

Fast-twitch muscle fibers, on the other hand, engender high levels of force for short periods. They're the ones we use for weight training. Conceivably, the difference between the two women's performances might have resulted from the fact that Keisha had more slow-twitch fibers while Pat had a higher proportion of the fast-twitch kind.

Another factor in strength training is the length of your muscles. Usually, long-limbed people have longer muscles, while short-limbed people have shorter muscles. But long-boned, long-muscled people are at a distinct disadvantage when it comes to lifting weights because their leverage isn't as good.

In the end, though, both Pat and Keisha realized that their differences did not matter all that much. Though Pat saw faster gains in strength training while Keisha made quicker progress in the cardio workouts, both women grew more fit and healthy, and each lost the weight she wanted to lose. Regardless of how gifted any of us is in one domain or the other, the Fat Flush Fitness Plan has us work on both—and both areas will improve from this balanced exercise.

So if you feel like comparing yourself to another woman you know, don't. Focus on your own body, your own progress, and your own pleasure in working out. No matter who reaches her goal before you or after you, the important thing is that you get there.

Using a Strength Ball

To proceed with phase 2 of the Fat Flush Fitness Plan, you'll need to buy a strength ball. A strength ball—also known as a medicine ball—is a weighted ball that comes in various styles and sizes. When you go shopping for one, you'll discover that the balls can weigh anywhere from 2 to 30 pounds, and they come in sizes ranging from a grapefruit to a basketball. For the Fat Flush Fitness Plan, we recommend getting a ball that's about two-thirds the size of a volleyball. For women, we recommend the 6-pound ball, and for men, the one that weighs 10 pounds. However, if you've been doing weight training or another type of upper-body exercise and you're more comfortable with a heavier ball, go for it. Women might use a ball weighing from 6 to 15 pounds, and men, from 10 to 20. Just don't overdo. Sustained work with a lighter ball is far more valuable than sporadic work with a heavier ball, and choosing a ball that's too heavy for you is not only demoralizing, it could lead to serious injury.

This is the rule of strength training: in order to get stronger, work with heavier weights and perform fewer repetitions; to promote endurance, use lighter weights and complete more repetitions. The goal of the workout is to increase muscle strength and improve fat-to-lean muscle mass ratio.[3]

By the way, don't confuse a strength ball with those large, inflatable balls on which you sit or roll. The strength ball is small enough to hold in your hand, with a rubber or polyurethane surface that is soft on your fingers. Its textured grip makes it easier to hold. Remember, too, that you're looking for the nonbounce type of strength ball. (For more on buying a strength ball, see Chapter 10.)

Strength balls provide weight resistance through a full range of motion. Working out with a strength ball helps tightens core muscles in your abdomen and back. Your core muscles are especially important because they stabilize your spine. Think of your core as a strong pole that links your lower and upper body. If you have a strong core, that creates a solid foundation for everything else you do.

You'll also be strengthening your shoulders, chest, arms, and legs. One of the greatest benefits of working out with a strength ball is increased flexibility.

If you haven't been exercising regularly, you may have noticed that you just don't bound up from your seat the way you used to, that as the weeks and months go by, you're discovering aches, pains, and stiffness in your lower back, knees, elbows, and neck. Using a strength ball will bring back muscle strength and flexibility, as the weight of the ball requires you to put your body through a wide range of motion while still exerting muscle control.

As we've mentioned, it's a good idea to have a workout outfit, a separate set of clothes that reminds you—and the others in your family—that this is your workout time. You don't need a separate strength training outfit, though. Feel free to wear the same clothing and shoes that you use for your rebounding or walking; just be sure that your clothes don't restrict your movements.

Your Cardio Workout: Phase 2

Even as you're adding strength training, phase 2 also has you increasing your cardio workout, ideally up to thirty minutes a day, followed by five minutes of cool-down stretches. If you can't do thirty minutes without becoming breathless or fatigued, start with twenty minutes and work your way up.

Remember that you must always warm up before your cardio workout—otherwise, you risk soreness, injury, and greater stiffness than you had before. So use your five-minute Sun Salutation to get the oxygen and blood flowing throughout your body and warming up your muscles.

Then, as you complete your cardio workout, use the last two minutes to lower your heart rate gradually, so the end of the workout serves as a preparation for cool-down/stretching.

If Your Cardio Workout Is Walking . . .

If you're walking, continue as before, walking briskly as you pump your arms and breathe deeply. Your goal is to walk thirty minutes without stopping or becoming so breathless you can't talk. If you can't manage that, start with what you *can* do—but do walk briskly, and do walk five days a week. Work your way up gradually to the full, brisk thirty minutes. You've got six weeks to be on phase 2, so you should be able to manage thirty minutes, five times a week, by then. If you're already able to walk thirty minutes easily, you can give yourself a further challenge if you choose; walk a bit longer, or maybe walk some hills for intensity.

If Your Cardio Workout Is Rebounding . . .

If you're rebounding, start this thirty-minute workout in phase 2. If you're not quite there, work your way up from a shorter workout—but exercise five days a week, even if you can only manage five, ten, or fifteen minutes. The daily exercise really makes a difference in your oxygen levels, blood flow, and general energy.

EXERCISE 1: WALK BOUNCE—FIVE MINUTES
1. Walk in place at an easy pace.
2. Allow your arms to hang loosely at your sides.

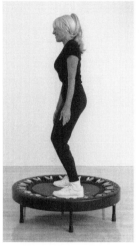

EXERCISE 2: FLAT BOUNCE—FIVE MINUTES
1. Start with your feet about twelve inches apart.
2. Keeping your feet on the surface, begin a small bouncing motion. At the height of your bounce, your legs will be straight; when you land, allow your knees to bend slightly.
3. Allow your arms to hang loosely at your sides.

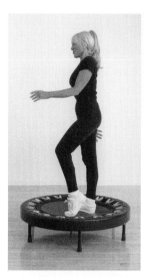

EXERCISE 3: MARCH BOUNCE—FIVE MINUTES
1. Raise your left heel, keeping your toes and right foot on the surface.
2. Swing your right arm forward and left arm back.
3. Repeat with your right heel and left arm.

EXERCISE 4: LYMPH ACTIVATOR BOUNCE—FIVE MINUTES
1. Start with both feet on the mat, arms at your sides. Use your arms and ankles to begin to bounce with your feet leaving the mat.
2. Increase the bounce until your feet are about three inches off the mat with your legs held straight.

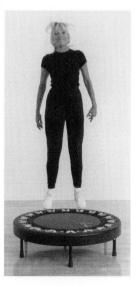

EXERCISE 5: MARCH BOUNCE—FIVE MINUTES
1. Follow instructions for exercise 3.

EXERCISE 6: WALK BOUNCE—FIVE MINUTES

1. Follow instructions for exercise 1. Remember to cool down for the last two minutes of the walk bounce.

Cool-Down Stretching After Your Cardio Workout: Phase 2

In phase 2 of the Fat Flush Fitness Plan, you will do thirty minutes of cardio five days a week. On two of those days, you'll add some weight training, and we've designed some special stretches to do at the end of the Strength Ball Workout. We can't stress this point too strongly—you *must* also do your cool-down stretches after your cardio workout! Otherwise, you risk aching muscles, stiff joints, and potential injury. Your goal is to become flexible, supple, and strong—and only your stretches will help you achieve it.

Coordinating Your Cardio and Strength Ball Workouts

If you're too tired to do a strength ball workout after thirty minutes of cardio, cut back your cardio workout to ten or fifteen minutes on the two days you do your strength training.

If you like, you can break up your workout, doing your cardio and strength training at different times. In that case, do a five-minute Sun Salutation warm-up before each workout, and then do five minutes of cool-down stretches after each workout. Use the stretches from phase 1 for the cardio cool-down, and the stretches from phase 2 for the strength ball cool-down.

Fat Flush Strength Ball Workout
Six-Week Schedule

We want you to take your time becoming accustomed to strength training. So we've constructed a program that gives you two weeks to get used to each workout level before gently nudging you up a notch.

Phase 2: Strength Ball Workout Six-Week Schedule

	EXERCISE	MUSCLE GROUP	REPS	SET
1	**Standing Ball Knee Raise**	quads, gluteals, abs	10*	1**
2	**Standing Ball Oblique Twist**	abs (obliques)	10*	1**
3	**Overhead Ball Squat**	quads, hamstrings, gluteals, upper body	10*	1**
4	**Standing Lunge/ Side Ball Pass**	buttocks, quads, calves, hamstrings, upper body	8 on left 8 on right	1**
5	**Ball Side Lunge**	buttocks, biceps	8 on left 8 on right	1
6	**Ball Trunk Rotation**	abs (obliques)	10*	1**
7	**Ball Over-Under**	abs, back	10	1
8	**Ball Overhead Crunch**	abs	12	1
9	**Ball Knee Twist**	abs, adductors, back	10*	1**

*Both right and left
**A set consists of an equal number of reps, both right and left

Your Strength Training Workout: Phase 2

EXERCISE 1: STANDING BALL KNEE RAISE

1. Stand with your feet slightly more than shoulder-width apart. Hold the ball both hands, arms extended over your head.
2. Bend and raise your right knee toward your right shoulder as far as possible, keeping your back straight.
3. At the same time, bring the ball down to your knee, touch your knee, and then lift your arms (holding the ball) back over your head as you lower your right knee to the starting position.

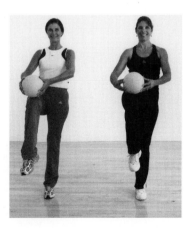

4. Repeat with the opposite side.
5. Repeat for a total of ten repetitions (reps), or one set.

Muscles targeted: quadriceps, hamstrings, abs.

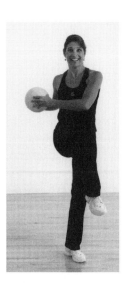

EXERCISE 2: STANDING BALL OBLIQUE TWIST

1. Stand with your feet slightly more than shoulder-width apart.
2. Bend and raise your right knee toward your left elbow, while you move your left elbow toward your right knee. The movement should twist your upper body toward the right and your lower body toward the left.
3. Return to the starting position and repeat with the opposite side.

Strength Training Do's and Don'ts

DO

- Warm up—always. If you start with your cardio workout, that's a terrific warm-up. If you want to do your cardio and your strength training at different times of day, do a five-minute Sun Salutation before each workout.

- Use good form. Don't arch your back or rock your body, which can cause injury as well as make the exercise less effective.

- Practice good posture to protect your lower back.

- Pick up the strength ball with your knees bent and your back straight.

DON'T

- Hold your breath while you exercise—it can increase your blood pressure.

- Move too quickly. A jerky movement can cause injury. And slowing down can help ensure that you're using the correct range of motion for each exercise.

4. Alternate one side and then the other, to equal one rep. Repeat for ten reps (one set).

Muscles targeted: abdominals (obliques)

EXERCISE 3: OVERHEAD BALL SQUAT

1. Stand with your feet shoulder-width apart.
2. Hold the ball over your head, arms extended, but slightly bent (not locked). Pull your abdominals in.
3. Bend your knees and lower your body as if sitting in a chair, with your weight slightly back on your heels. As you do so, bring the ball down to the top of your thighs, which should be parallel to the floor. If your knees move forward over your toes, you've gone too far
4. Straighten your legs as you stand back up, but don't lock your knees at the top of the movement. Be sure that your heels remain on the floor at all times.
5. As you stand back up, bring the ball over your head, arms slightly bent. Inhale as you lower and exhale as you raise the ball.
6. Repeat for a total of eight reps (one set).

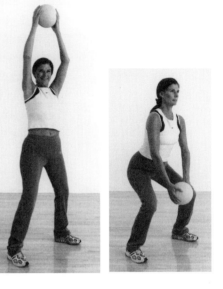

Muscles targeted: quadriceps, hamstrings, gluteals, upper body

EXERCISE 4: STANDING LUNGE/SIDE BALL PASS

1. Stand with your left leg forward a stride ahead of the right leg—lift your right heel (at 12 o'clock and 6 o'clock). Face right, holding ball in both hands at hip level.
2. Lower your body until the upper left leg is parllel to the floor, keeping your left knee aligned with yur left ankle. ,Bring the ball to the front, resting on your left knee.
3. Rise and face right, holding the ball in both hands at hip level as in position 1.
4. Repeat for a total of eight reps (one set),

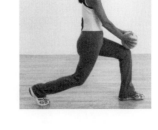

5. Repeat series with your right leg forward, facing left, the ball in both hands at hip level. Do a total of eight reps (one set).

Muscles targeted: buttocks, quadriceps, hamstrings, calves, upper body

EXERCISE 5: BALL SIDE LUNGE

1. From the start position, stand with your feet shoulder-width apart, legs straight, abdominals in, and ball held at mid-torso in front of you with both elbows bent.
2. Pulling your abdominals in, take a large sidestep (to 9 o'clock) with your left foot, toes pointing slightly outward, bending your left knee so it stays in line with your left ankle. (If your bent knee goes past your toes or rotates in, this can stress knee ligaments and tendons.) Your right leg should be straight, foot flat on the floor with toes pointing forward, and your body centered between both legs.

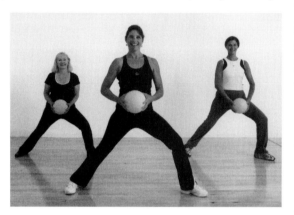

3. As you take your large step to the side, lower the ball in front of you (keep your eyes focused straight ahead, so you do not turn your body).
4. Push off your left foot, lift the ball to your chest (biceps curl), and bring your feet together, back to the starting position.
5. Return to the starting position. Inhale as you step out and lower the ball, and exhale as you lift the ball and return to the starting position.
6. Repeat for a total of eight reps (one set).
7. Now do the exercise again on the right side, taking a large sidestep to the right as you lower the ball.
8. Lift the ball and return to the starting position.
9. Repeat for eight reps (one set).

Muscles targeted: buttocks, biceps

EXERCISE 6: BALL TRUNK ROTATION

1. Sit on the floor with your legs spread apart in front of you (in a **V**) and the ball between your legs.
2. Pick up the ball with both hands, rotate your upper body to the left and tap the ball on the floor, outside your leg

3. Twist back to the right, across the center position, and tap the ball on the floor to the right, outside your leg. Try to make as full a circle as you can, aiming for the same spot on the floor from left to right. Do not roll your hips or buttocks off the ground; only your upper body should be rotating. When you have tapped the floor on both the left and the right sides, you have completed one rep.

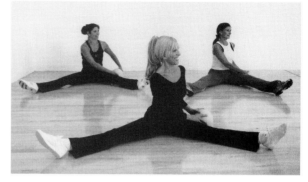

4. Repeat for a total of ten reps (one set).

Muscles targeted: abs (obliques)

EXERCISE 7: BALL OVER-UNDER

1. Sit on the floor with your legs spread apart in front of you (in a **V**) and the ball between your legs. Pull in your abdominals and sit up straight.
2. Lift your left leg and pass the ball under it from the inside.
3. Pass the ball over the top of your left leg, under your right leg from the inside, and over the top of your right leg (so the ball makes a figure eight around your legs).
4. Repeat ten reps, or ten figure eights (one set).

Muscles targeted: abs, back

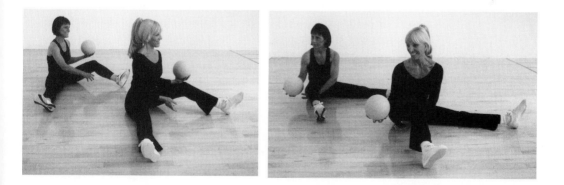

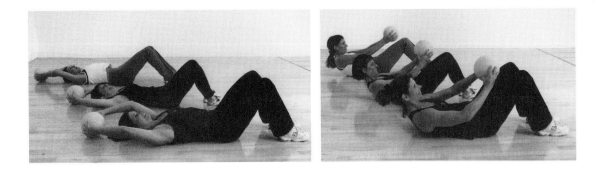

EXERCISE 8: BALL OVERHEAD CRUNCH

1. Lie on your back with your knees bent, feet flat on the floor. Hold the ball with both hands.
2. Lift your arms over your head, arms slightly bent and in line with your ears. Pull in your abdominals to assure that your spine is on the floor.
3. Curl your torso upward, moving as one unit, bringing your shoulder blades off the floor as your ribs and hips come closer together. Do not arch your back. Pause .
4. Lower your torso to the starting position with your arms over your head.
5. Repeat for a total of twelve reps (one set).

Muscles targeted: abdominals

EXERCISE 9: BALL KNEE TWIST

1. Lie flat on your back on the floor, knees bent, with your arms straight out to the sides. Pull in your abdominals.
2. Lift your knees up and place the ball between your knees. Press inward to secure the ball in place.

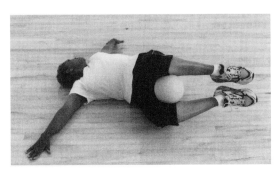

3. With a slow and controlled movement, lower your knees toward the left side to a count of four, keeping your shoulders and back flat on the floor .
4. Return your knees to the center position (to a count of four) over your hips; then lower them to the right (for four counts).

The Fat Flush Fitness Plan

5. Return your knees to the center position. When you have lowered your knees to the left, center, and right, you have completed one rep.
6. Repeat for a total of ten reps (one set).

Muscles targeted: adductors, abs, back

Strength Ball Cool-Down Stretches: Phase 2

You've already learned the cool-down stretches to do after your cardio workout, but you'll want a different set of stretches to ease out of your strength ball workout. We've designed this set of stretches specifically for the muscles that you use while working with the strength ball.

Benefits of the Strength Ball Routine
- Improves function of your lymphatic system

- Raises your metabolic rate

- Increases muscle strength and endurance

- Improves your posture

- Reduces your risk of osteoporosis

- Elevates your mood

- Helps with balance and coordination

The Correct Way to Stretch

Remember to breathe deeply, to move into each stretch slowly, and never to force yourself beyond what seems comfortable. Avoid bouncing during a stretch, which shortens the muscles. Instead, find a comfortable position and then breathe into it as you hold the stretch—almost as if your body is working on its own.

EXERCISE 1: FLOOR ELONGATION STRETCH
1. Lie on your back with your arms and fingers extended overhead.
2. Straighten your legs and extend your toes like you are trying to be as tall as possible. You should now be reaching in both directions, as if someone is pulling you from both the top and the bottom.
3. Stretch for five seconds, and then relax.
4. Repeat.

Tip: Completing this elongation stretch at least four times will reduce tension and tightness in your spine; it will stretch the spine and your abdominal muscles, as well as your shoulders, arms, ankles, and feet.

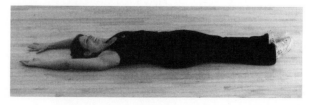

EXERCISE 2: ALTERNATE KNEE TO CHEST STRETCH

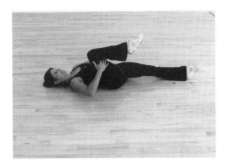

1. Stay in the relaxed elongated stretch position from exercise 1 and gently pull your right knee toward your chest. Keep your upper body as well as the back of your head on the floor if possible, but don't strain. If you can't do it with your head down, use a small pillow under your head. Keep your left leg as straight as possible without locking your knee.
2. Hold this position for twenty seconds.
3. Repeat the stretch, this time bringing your left knee to your chest and extending your right leg.

Tip: This stretch will stretch your back and hamstrings.

EXERCISE 3: LOWER BACK STRETCH, FLOOR VERSION

1. Start in the elongated stretch position (relaxed), but this time place your arms out to the sides (you should be in a **T** position).
2. Bend your right leg and cross it over your left leg (which is extended with the knee slightly bent).
3. Bring your left arm down and gently pull your right knee to the left as far as you comfortably can

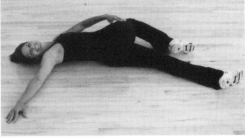

4. Turn your head to the right, and try to keep both shoulders on the ground. Hold for thirty seconds.
5. Repeat the stretch, this time crossing your left leg over your right.

Tip: This stretch is for your back and your gluteal muscles.

EXERCISE 4: STANDING CHEST EXPANSION

1. Stand tall and bring your arms behind you, clasping one hand inside the other.
2. Lift your chest and raise your arms slightly. You should feel the

stretch across your chest and down the back of your arms. Try to resist arching your back as you lift your arms upward, and be sure not to force your arms up higher than is comfortable. Keep your shoulders low and relaxed.

3. Hold the stretch for fifteen seconds. Do this stretch at least twice.

Tip: This stretch is for your shoulders, chest, and arms and will help your posture immeasurably.

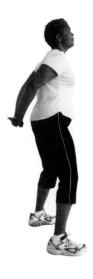

EXERCISE 5: BACK EXPANSION

1. Stand tall, knees slightly bent, feet shoulder-width apart. Lift your arms in front of you to shoulder height. Clasp one hand in the other.
2. Drop your head toward your chest, round your back, and pull your abdominals in while you press your hips forward, so that you create a **C** shape with your body.
3. Stretch your arms forward, which will move your shoulder blades apart. Keep your abdominal muscles pulled in to protect your back. Keep your shoulders low and relaxed.
4. Lean forward only as far as you can without losing your balance.
5. Hold the stretch for fifteen seconds. Do this stretch twice.

Tip: This stretch is for your back, shoulders, and arms.

EXERCISE 6: NECK STRETCH

1. Stand tall, knees slightly bent, feet shoulder-width apart. Keep your shoulders level. Pull your chin back and in, and keep the top of your head toward the ceiling; your arms should be behind you.
2. To stretch the right side of your neck, slowly lean your head to the left side (left ear lobe toward the left shoulder—be sure not to rotate your neck).
3. With your left hand, gently pull your right arm down and across your back to the left.
4. Hold for fifteen seconds, breathing evenly as you hold the stretch.
5. Move your head gently back to center and repeat the stretch on your right side (stretching out the left side of the neck). This time, lean your head to the right side (right ear lobe toward the right shoulder—do not rotate your neck) and use your right hand to gently pull your left arm down and across your back to the right. Hold for fifteen seconds.
6. Do both sides twice, alternating right and left.

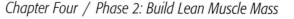

Tips for Making It Through Phase 2

- When you visualize working out, imagine doing the part you enjoy most. When we have to schedule something into a busy day, we tend to think of how difficult it will be to find the time. Focus on the segment of the workout you love most—the slow stretching of the Sun Salutation, the carefree bouncing on your rebounder, even the pleasant glow when your workout is over. Whatever your favorite part is it will encourage you to find the time to work out.

- Give yourself a day or two to learn the strength training and stretching routines. If you haven't worked out with a strength ball before, it can take a while to get comfortable. Just relax—you've got six weeks! Walk through each routine once slowly, consulting this book, to make sure you understand the exercise. Then try a few reps. If you don't have time to do the full workout for the first few days, don't worry. It's more important that you get comfortable with each exercise.

- When you get halfway through phase 2, buy yourself something new. Even if you're waiting to replenish your wardrobe until you've achieved your entire weight goal, splurge on something at this point. You'll be delighted to see how differently you wear clothes now that you're slimmer, more toned, and standing up straighter. For extra motivation points, dare yourself to buy a type of outfit you might have avoided previously—something sexier, more revealing, or more comfortable than you were able to wear before.

- Be good to yourself—*especially* when you've missed a day of working out or eaten something not on the plan. Beating yourself up and feeling terrible will only make it harder to continue. The most successful people in life are those who start from where they are at the present moment, letting go of the past and moving forward with a clean slate. If there's a reason you slipped that you can correct, then by all means, make the change. Maybe you didn't buy enough healthy snacks for yourself and so you fell prey to your husband's potato chips, or perhaps you convinced yourself that you had time for a workout *and* a trip to the shoe store when you knew in your heart that you could only do one or the other. Figure out how to avoid that mistake in the future—but then let it go. Tomorrow is *always* another day. Stressing, obsessing, and feeling blue will only raise your cortisol levels!

Rest and Renewal Days: Phase 2

As always, you get two free days in phase 2 to do whatever you like. After five days of exercise, you'll feel more alert mentally and energized physically. Ask yourself what will restore your mind, body, and spirit, and then go for it.

Lots of women like to start each rest and renewal day with the Sun Salutation. We think it's an ideal way to get your blood flowing and to stay connected to your physical self—but it's your choice. You might find yourself drawn to some vigorous activity, such as hiking, biking, or working in the garden. Or you may luxuriate in some time to read a book, listen to music, or take yourself to a movie. The point is that it's your choice—so enjoy!

Somewhere in your seven-day week, you need to schedule in three aromatherapy baths and two brief sessions of dry-brush massage. Check out Chapter 7 for more detail on these relaxing treats. And remember—now that you're building up lean muscle mass, you're burning calories even when you're soaking in the tub!

Phase 2 Workout Calendar

Time for your workout calendar again! We suggest that you fill this out in two-week segments, so you can see how the new, expanded phase 2 workout schedule best fits into your own schedule. Some women, however, find doing the calendar one week at a time more helpful. Make sure that you do plan ahead, so that you can give your workout time as much priority as any other aspect of your busy life. And don't forget your eight hours of sleep and time for your journal. Just tell yourself that the time you invest in sleep and journaling will more than be made up in the extra energy you have as you become more fit.

My Fat Flush Fitness Plan Workout Calendar: Phase 2 (weeks 1 and 2)

	Monday	Tuesday	Wednesday	Thursday	Friday	Saturday	Sunday
8 A.M.							
9 A.M.							
10 A.M.							
11 A.M.							
Noon							
1 P.M.							
2 P.M.							
3 P.M.							
4 P.M.							
5 P.M.							
6 P.M.							
7 P.M.							
8 P.M.							
9 P.M.							
10 P.M.							

The Fat Flush Fitness Plan

My Fat Flush Fitness Plan Workout Calendar: Phase 2 (weeks 3 and 4)

	Monday	Tuesday	Wednesday	Thursday	Friday	Saturday	Sunday
8 A.M.							
9 A.M.							
10 A.M.							
11 A.M.							
Noon							
1 P.M.							
2 P.M.							
3 P.M.							
4 P.M.							
5 P.M.							
6 P.M.							
7 P.M.							
8 P.M.							
9 P.M.							
10 P.M.							

My Fat Flush Fitness Plan Workout Calendar: Phase 2 (weeks 5 and 6)

	Monday	Tuesday	Wednesday	Thursday	Friday	Saturday	Sunday
8 A.M.							
9 A.M.							
10 A.M.							
11 A.M.							
Noon							
1 P.M.							
2 P.M.							
3 P.M.							
4 P.M.							
5 P.M.							
6 P.M.							
7 P.M.							
8 P.M.							
9 P.M.							
10 P.M.							

My Fat Flush Fitness Plan Workout Calendar: Phase 2 (weeks 7 and 8)

	Monday	Tuesday	Wednesday	Thursday	Friday	Saturday	Sunday
8 A.M.							
9 A.M.							
10 A.M.							
11 A.M.							
Noon							
1 P.M.							
2 P.M.							
3 P.M.							
4 P.M.							
5 P.M.							
6 P.M.							
7 P.M.							
8 P.M.							
9 P.M.							
10 P.M.							

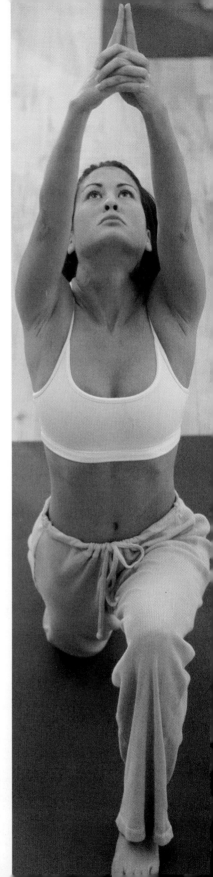

5
Phase 3: Lymph-Fit/ Compound Strength and Stretching Plan

The Fat Flush Fitness Plan—Phase 3: FOUR WEEKS
- Sun Salutation—five minutes, five days a week

- Rebounding or a brisk walk—forty minutes, five days a week
     Three days a week followed by cool-down stretches—five minutes
     Two days a week followed by Lymph-Fit workout/cool-down stretches—
     twenty five minutes

- Lymphatic massage—half an hour, once a week

- Dry-brush massage—five minutes, twice a week

- Aromatherapy bath—twenty minutes, three times a week

Congratulations! You've now moved on to phase 3 of the Fat Flush Fitness Plan. This portion of the plan increases your cardio workout and adds a unique set of exercises we call the Lymph-Fit/Compound Strength and Stretching workout. The Lymph-Fit/Compound Strength and Stretching workout will improve your posture; aid you to continue (and maintain) losing fat from your hip, thighs, and tummy; and—as the name suggests—help keep your lymph flowing. Some women have even found that the Lymph-Fit/Compound Strength and Stretching workout enables them to get rid of the remaining traces of cellulite—the rough and dimply texture of the hips and thighs that many doctors believe cannot be eliminated—even faster. We can't guarantee that you'll be cellulite free—but we can tell you that dozens of women have had that experience. (For more about cellulite, check out Chapter 8.)

You might be wondering what happened to the strength training portion of your workout. Don't worry. Between the increased cardio activity and the new Lymph-Fit/Compound Strength and Stretching component, you'll be using your own body's weight as resistance, building strength as you continue to develop lean muscle mass. This phase, too, features a combination of dry-brushing and lymphatic massage, for the final push to cleanse and detoxify your lymph.

So let's get started! Many women find that phase 3 of both the eating plan and the exercise plan is the most satisfying component of all.

Adding the Lymph-Fit/Compound Strength and Stretching Workout to Your Routine

The Lymph-Fit/Compound Strength and Stretching workout is all about standing up straight, opening your chest, breathing deeply, and strengthening the muscles of the trunk, or core, of the body. It is the muscles of the core—abdomen, chest, and back—that stabilize the rest of the body. Good posture and deep breathing are the best possible medicines for your lymphatic system. Standing up straight allows lymph to flow through the inguinal canal at your groin and the thoracic duct next to your heart. Deep breathing creates a negative pressure in your chest that helps pull lymph through to the thoracic duct, on the way to its final cleansing. You'll be doing the Lymph-Fit/Compound Strength and Stretching workout in your bare feet. Pointing your toes and working in bare feet are also excellent for helping lymph drain from the hips, thighs, and calves. Who knew that good posture was so good for your health?

Perhaps more important, we've learned through working with thousands of women that good posture makes a surprising difference in the way you feel about yourself. Women report a new sense of pride and pleasure in themselves, a new comfort in taking up space and making their presence felt. Of course, some of that is due to their new physical self-confidence as they have lost weight and gained fitness. But some of it is the powerful statement that is made—to ourselves as well as to others—when we simply stand up straight.

One of our favorite comments is the one that Cecily, a sweet, shy, and extremely attractive woman in her early forties, made. "I've basically been looking down my whole life, and I didn't realize it," Cecily told Joanie. "I always associated holding myself upright with phony posturing. I didn't realize you could stand tall and still look natural."

Sounds good, doesn't it? So let's get started on phase 3.

Your Cardio Workout: Phase 3

As in phase 2, you'll be doing cardio five days a week, and by now that should be—pardon the expression—a piece of cake. By this time, too, you should be able to up your cardio to the forty minutes we've allotted to phase 3. Three times a week you'll do cool-down stretches after your cardio—the same cool-down stretches you've done in phases 1 and 2. Twice a week you'll follow up your cardio with the Lymph-Fit/Compound Strength and Stretching workout, followed in turn by its own special set of stretches.

As always, you'll want to use your Sun Salutation to warm up for your cardio workout, and to use the last two minutes of your workout to gradually decrease your speed or intensity, lowering your heart rate and preparing for the cool-down period. Your goal is to push yourself without overdoing it—getting right up to the edge of exertion without creating excessive fatigue.

If Your Cardio Workout Is Walking . . .

If you're walking, do exactly what you've been doing—just do it for forty minutes instead of thirty. You're welcome to add some hills or steep terrain to up the ante, but don't choose any type of walking where you have to struggle.

Benefits of Phase 3

- Your lymphatic flow will be increased.

- Your circulation will improve.

- You will strengthen core muscles.

- You will increase your flexibility.

- You will continue to lose weight and gain muscle tone.

- Your posture will improve dramatically.

- You'll improve your balance and coordination.

- You'll be less prone to fatigue.

- You'll be calmer and more serene.

Your goal is brisk, continuous movement, ideally supported by deep breathing. If you can't talk at all, you're moving too fast. If you can carry on a long, unbroken conversation, you're moving too slow. Other than that, it's all up to you. Enjoy!

If Your Cardio Workout Is Rebounding . . .

If you're rebounding, your phase 3 goal is to bounce for forty minutes. Here's the sequence of exercises you can use. Remember to slow down and cool down as you enter the last few minutes.

EXERCISE 1: WALK BOUNCE—FIVE MINUTES
1. Walk in place at an easy pace.
2. Allow your arms to hang loosely at your sides.

EXERCISE 2: FLAT BOUNCE—FIVE MINUTES
1. Start with your feet about twelve inches apart.
2. Keep your feet on the surface and begin a small bouncing motion. At the height of your bounce, your legs will be straight; when you land, allow your knees to bend slightly.

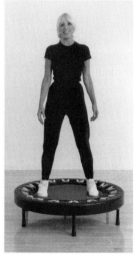

3. Allow your arms to hang loosely at your sides.

EXERCISE 3: MARCH BOUNCE WITH HIGH KNEES—FIVE MINUTES
1. March in place, bringing your knees up as high as you can without losing your balance.
2. Swing your right arm forward and left arm back, in opposition to your knees.

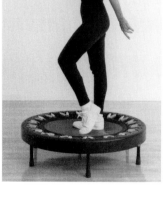

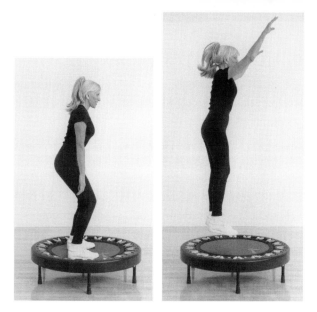

EXERCISE 4: STRENGTH BOUNCE—FIVE MINUTES

1. Bend your knees and then push off, straightening both knees as you go up.
2. Swing both arms upward at the same time
3. Bend your knees as you land and your arms come down.

EXERCISE 5: KICK BOUNCE—FIVE MINUTES

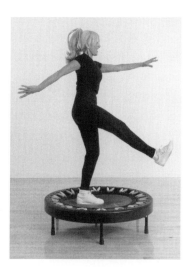

1. With your feet together, bounce once.
2. As you come up, kick the right leg straight out in front of you. Bring it back as you again bounce on both feet and then alternate by kicking the left leg straight out in front of you (kick—bounce—kick—bounce—kick—bounce).
3. Swing your arms in opposition to your legs.

EXERCISE 6: MARCH BOUNCE—FIVE MINUTES

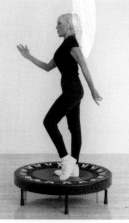

1. Raise your left heel, keeping your toes and right foot on the surface.
2. Swing your right arm forward and left arm back.
3. Repeat with your right heel and left arm .

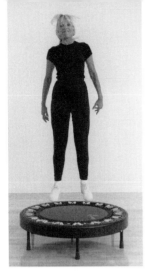

EXERCISE 7: LYMPH ACTIVATOR BOUNCE—FIVE MINUTES

1. Start with both feet on the mat, arms to your sides. Use your arms and ankles to begin to bounce with your feet just barely leaving the mat .
2. Increase the bounce until your feet are about three inches off the mat, with your legs held straight(see Figure 5.6).

EXERCISE 8: WALK BOUNCE—FIVE MINUTES

Repeat the Walk Bounce at a gradually decreasing intensity as you start to cool down.

Cool-Down Stretching After Your Cardio Workout: Phase 3

By now you should be well aware of how good stretching is for you—and how good it makes you feel! On the two days that you add the Lymph-Fit/Compound Strength and Stretching workout, you'll finish up your workout with some special Lymph-Fit stretching. But on the three days that you're doing only cardio, go back to the five-minute stretches that you learned in phase 1.

Think *flexible*—and think of how much easier it's suddenly become to reach for something on a high shelf or to bend down and look for your shoes beneath the bed! That comes from stretching—so make sure you don't skip even a single stretch. If you're running short on time, cut five minutes from your cardio—but never, never cut back on your stretching time. With all we've learned after decades of working in the nutrition and fitness fields, that may well be the most important advice we'll ever give you.

Coordinating Your Cardio and Lymph-Fit/ Compound Strength and Stretching Workouts

If you're too tired to do a Lymph-Fit workout after forty minutes of cardio, cut back to a ten- or fifteen-minute cardio workout on the two days you do your Lymph-Fit workout. If you go right from cardio to the Lymph-Fit workout, you can wait to do your cool-down stretches after the entire workout is finished—and we've designed some special stretches specifically for that workout.

If you want to do your cardio and Lymph-Fit workout at different times of the day, we recommend you do a five-minute Sun Salutation warm-up before each workout; also do five minutes of cool-down stretches after each workout. Use the stretches from phase 1 for the cardio cool-down, and the stretches from phase 3 for the Lymph-Fit cool-down.

Your goal, of course, is to do the full phase 3 workout, and eventually you will be strong enough to do so. If you're not quite there, we suggest making a schedule in which you add five minutes to your cardio workout each week. Or, if you prefer, add one minute to your cardio workout each day. Either way, you should soon be doing the full forty-minute cardio workout, followed by the Lymph-Fit/Compound Strength and Stretching workout twice a week. Congratulations on achieving such a significant level of fitness!

The Lymph-Fit/Compound Strength and Stretching Workout: Promoting the Flow of Lymph

The Fat Flush Lymph-Fit/Compound Strength and Stretching workout has been specifically created for the Fat Flush Fitness Plan to improve the movement of lymphatic fluid. As we discussed in Chapter 1, there's no organ to pump the lymph through the body—instead, the lymphatic system relies on breathing, muscular contractions, and the movement of organs surrounding the lymphatic vessels to push the fluids to their destination. So this workout focuses on breathing and lymph-friendly muscle movements. It also will help improve your posture, which in turn will open your chest, promote lymph movement into the thoracic duct, and free up the area around the inguinal canal.[1]

Your Posture and Your Health

As mentioned, poor posture compromises the inguinal canal—the narrow channel in the groin through which lymph vessels and veins pass as they drain away the fluid from the legs. Although covered by a tough coating of ligament, the inguinal canal can be compromised by outside pressure such as tight clothing, excess weight, sitting for long periods of time, and—you guessed it—poor posture.

All sorts of health problems result when the inguinal canal is compromised. Lymph vessels and veins aren't able to drain fluid properly from the

Fat Flush Lymph-Fit/Compound Strength and Stretching Workout Do's and Don'ts

DO

- Wear well-fitting clothing that's not too tight.

- Go barefoot.

- Find a room with carpeting or use a mat.

- Have a straight-backed chair available for the standing exercises.

- Drink some water before and after you exercise to stay hydrated, but avoid drinking while you work out, especially cold or iced water—you might get a cramp.

- Stand tall and pull in your abdominals, keeping your head up and your shoulders back. Imagine a string pulling you up from the top of your head so that everything lifts up.

- Breathe deeply while you work out.

- Use slow, controlled movements.

DON'T

- Hold your breath—it can increase your blood pressure.

- Slouch.

- Rush the exercise.

legs. Tissue fluids begin binding to fat cells, which in turn swell up. The swelling leads to still more lymphatic fluid backup and in many cases the development of cellulite, as we'll discuss further in Chapter 8.

The key to freeing up the inguinal canal is posture. Standing with poor posture—abdominal area sticking out, lower spine rounded—can compress the inguinal canal. Likewise, weak abdominal muscles compromise the function of the thoracoabdominal pump, which despite its name is not a pump, but a channel through which the lymph passes on its way through the body. When this pump isn't working properly, the result can be fluid retention in the legs and buttocks—and still more cellulite.[2]

On the other hand, good posture—pulling in your abs and aligning your spine—takes the pressure off the inguinal canal and allows your lymph to flow freely. By the same token, strengthening the abdominal muscles through good posture and exercise allows the thoracoabdominal pump to do its job of returning venous blood and lymph to general circulation.

Good posture provides lots of other health benefits, too. When your spine is straight and your back and abdominal muscles are toned and firm, you minimize strain on all your muscles, ligaments, bones, and joints. Standing with poor posture tends to compress the internal organs, while good posture frees them up. Likewise, good posture means that blood as well as lymph can flow freely, so that your body functions at its best.

Lots of women tell us that after they improve their posture with the Lymph-Fit/Compound Strength and Stretching workout, little aches and pains in their necks, shoulders, upper backs, and lower backs suddenly disappear. They also report new, healthy surges of energy—perhaps because the bundle of nerves running up and down the spine is unblocked so that neurochemical messages can flow freely.

Working Barefoot

Although we advise you to wear good, supportive shoes during all other phases of the Fat Flush Fitness Plan, you need to go barefoot during the Lymph-Fit/Compound Strength and Stretching workout. This allows you to take full advantage of the plantar fascia reflex. The plantar fascia is the core of fibrous tissue running between the heel of your foot and the base of your toes. This bundle of tissue contains many receptors which, when stimulated, seem to encourage lymph flow. Gentle movements of your feet, such as pointing your toes, also improve lymphatic flow up your legs. Perhaps that's why dancers have such pretty legs!

Strengthen and Lengthen Your Muscles

Besides helping to improve your posture and giving your feet a workout, the exercises in the Lymph-Fit/Compound Strength and Stretching workout target your lower-body muscles: hips, buttocks, and legs, as well as lower back and abdominal muscles. And the workout combines strengthening and stretching. This workout will help you become more flexible by working joints, ligaments, tendons, and connective tissue.

The Lymph-Fit/Compound Strength and Stretching Workout: Phase 3

Remember to warm up before doing these exercises. You can either do them immediately after your cardio workout, or following a five-minute Sun Salutation. But do *not* do them with cold muscles.

Marching In Place

1. Lift your knees to your chest as you march in place, swinging the opposite arms forward and back—left knee up, right arm forward, and vice versa. Keep your arms straight and toes pointed.
2. Focus carefully on proper posture throughout the movement, pulling in your abs, tightening your buttocks, and bringing each knee up to your chest. If you remember to imagine the string pulling you up from the top of your head, this will help you keep in proper alignment.
3. March with each knee for 150 counts (or 300 total steps).

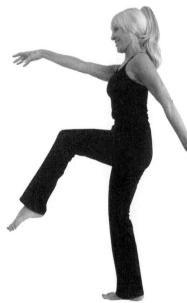

Hip Circle

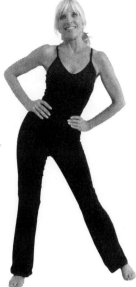

1. Place your hands on your hips and stand with your feet shoulder-width apart.
2. Bring your hips forward and try to make a perfect circle, as if you were standing in a barrel and trying to touch the sides with your body. As you do this, keep your head and shoulders relatively still, as you want to focus on moving your hips only.
3. Repeat four times in each direction.

Lymph-Fit Part 1: Standing Series

Do all the standing exercises in part 1 using a straight-backed chair.

EXERCISE 1: STRAIGHT LEG RAISE—FRONT

1. Turn sideways so your left side is next to the back of the chair. Hold onto the chair with your left hand. Keep your legs straight.
2. Take your right foot, pointing the toe, and raise your right leg straight in front of you as high as you can; the other leg can be slightly bent. Do not arch your back and do not raise your leg higher than is comfortable. Inhale and tighten the abdominal muscles as you bring your leg up.
3. Holding your right leg at the comfortable height, with toes pointed, do ten small lifts.
4. Exhale, release the tension, and lower the right leg to the floor.
5. Do one set of ten reps. As you become more familiar with the exercise, work up to three sets.

EXERCISE 2: STRAIGHT LEG RAISE—BACK

1. Use the same position as in exercise 1 with your left side next to the back of the chair.
2. Inhale and tighten your abdominal muscles.
3. Lift your right leg straight behind you, keeping your toes pointed. You may only be able to lift it a few inches—that's okay).
4. Breathe normally and then, as you did before, do ten small lifts.
5. Exhale, release the tension, and lower the right leg to the floor.
6. Do one set of ten reps. Try to work up to three sets.

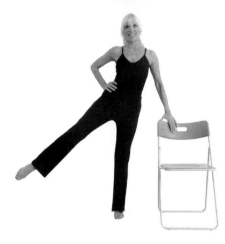

EXERCISE 3: STRAIGHT LEG RAISE—SIDE

1. Use the same position as in exercise 1, with your left side next to the back of the chair.
2. Inhale and tighten your abdominal muscles.
3. Lift your right leg straight out to the side, pointing your toes, but without turning your leg. Raise the leg as high as is comfortable. Keep your outer thigh and the outside of your foot toward the ceiling as you lift.
4. Breathe normally and do ten small lifts.
5. Exhale as you lower your leg to the floor. Try to work up to three sets.

EXERCISE 4: PLIÉ SQUAT

1. Stand facing the back of the chair with your legs straight and your feet a little more than shoulder-width apart, toes turned out slightly. Hold the back of the chair with both hands.
2. Inhale and tighten your abdominal muscles.
3. Exhale, bend your knees, and lower your hips to a 90-degree angle (no more) for four counts. (Check to be sure that your knees do not go past the end of your toes or your hips below your knees. You should still be able to see your feet if you are lined up correctly. If not, you have come down too low in your plié or your stance is not wide enough.)
4. Squeeze your inner thighs as you inhale and come back up in four counts.
5. Do one set of ten reps. Work your way up to two sets.

REPEAT EXERCISE 1 . . .
   raising the left leg.

REPEAT EXERCISE 2 . . .
   raising the left leg.

REPEAT EXERCISE 3 . . .
   raising the left leg.

REPEAT EXERCISE 4 . . .
   the plié squat.

TRANSITION TO FLOOR SERIES

Stand and repeat the Hip Circle on page 113. This will keep your circulation going and also loosen up your shoulders and hips.

Lymph-Fit Part 2: Floor Series

Be sure to do this series on a carpeted floor or a mat, not on a hard floor.

EXERCISE 9: LYING LEG RAISE–SIDE

1. Lie on your left side on the floor with your left leg slightly bent underneath, but your top leg straight. Your left arm is extended over your head. You can either rest your head on your left arm or slightly in front of it. Put your right hand on the floor in front of your chest for support.
2. Keeping your body still, inhale, pull in your abdominals, and squeeze your buttocks.

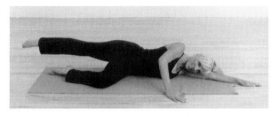 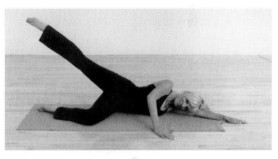

3. Pointing your toes, lift your right leg (outer thigh and the side of your foot facing the ceiling), breathe normally, and do ten small lifts. Exhale as you lower your leg.
4. Do one set of ten reps. Work your way up to three sets.

EXERCISE 10: LYING LEG COMBINATION–LEFT SIDE

1. Use the same position as in exercise 9: left side on the floor, left leg slightly bent underneath, and top leg straight. Inhale and make sure your body is in proper alignment.
2. Exhale for four counts as you lift your right leg straight out in front of your body; keep your toes pointed.

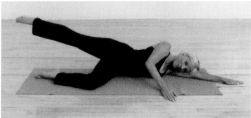

3. Inhale for four counts as you bend your right leg and bring it back so that your knees are together.
4. Exhale for four counts and extend the right leg straight behind you, pointing the toes . Pay careful attention not to roll out of your original position; only the leg should move. Imagine you're doing this under your bed so that you don't lift your leg higher as it goes behind you and out of sight. Inhale for four counts as you bring your leg back to the starting position. Don't rush; use your entire four counts.

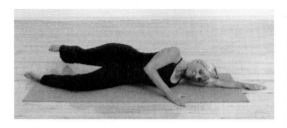

5. Do one set of ten reps.

EXERCISE 11: LYING LEG COMBINATION—RIGHT SIDE

Repeat exercise 10 using your left leg, with your right side on the floor, right leg slightly bent underneath, and top leg straight.

EXERCISE 12: STRAIGHT LEG KICKBACK

1. Position yourself on your hands and knees. Bring your hands together, palms down, and rest your forehead on the backs of your hands.
2. Pull in your abdominals and tighten your buttocks.
3. Point your toes and inhale for four counts as you bring your right knee to your chest.
4. Exhale for four counts as you extend your leg back and up as far as you can. Repeat with the right leg for one set of ten reps.
5. Do the exercise with your left leg for one set of ten reps. Work up to two sets per leg.

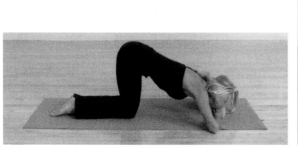
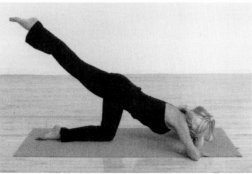

The Fat Flush Fitness Plan

EXERCISE 13: BENT LEG LIFT KICKS

1. Lie on your back with your hands palms down at your sides, legs straight up, and toes pointed. Pull in the abdominals so your back is flat on the floor with no arching.

2. Keeping your toes pointed, inhale and bend your right leg so your toes are pointing toward the floor (take four counts).

3. Breathing normally, do ten small lift kicks with your right leg while keeping the knee bent. Do one set of ten reps.

4. Exhale (for four counts) and bring your right leg up to the starting position.

5. Bend the left leg and repeat the exercise with your left leg for one set of ten reps. Return to the starting position. Flex both feet.

6. Inhale and bend your right leg (for four counts) and do ten small lift kicks while keeping your knee bent. Do one set of ten reps.

7. Exhale and bring your right leg up to the starting position (for four counts), keeping your feet flexed.

8. Bend the left leg and repeat the exercise with the left leg for one set of ten reps. Return to the starting position.

9. Repeat steps 1 through 6, keeping your toes pointed and remembering to exhale for four counts and inhale for four counts.

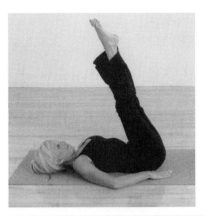

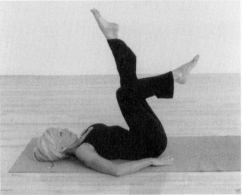

Lymph-Fit Cool-Down Stretches: Phase 3

You've been familiar with stretching for a few weeks now, so you'll understand why we've designed a special set of stretches to relax and loosen muscles after the Lymph-Fit/Compound Strength and Stretching workout.

Stretching Correctly

As always, remember to breathe deeply, into the stretch, to allow your muscles to relax and stretch as far as possible without excessive effort. And, of course, no bouncing—it only makes your muscles shorter and tighter, and you're going for long and loose.

EXERCISE 1: LOWER BACK STRETCH

1. While still on your back, after exercise 13, hug your knees and pull them into your chest. Continue to press your lumbar spine against the ground.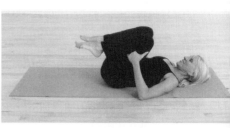
2. Roll your body gently from side to side, right to left, breathing slowly and deeply.
3. Repeat at least four or five times, holding the stretch to the side as long as you feel comfortable. This is a great way to release tension in the lower back.

EXERCISE 2: SPINAL STRETCH

1. While still on your back, put your arms out to the sides (like a **T**) with your palms down.
2. Exhale and pull your legs up, knees together, and slowly lower them to the right until your knees touch the floor (for four counts). Turn your head to the left, making sure your shoulders, upper back, and arms are flat on the floor.
3. Inhale for four counts and exhale for four counts; repeat.
4. Slowly return your knees to the center position.
5. Exhale and slowly lower your legs to the left side until your knees touch the floor on the left. Turn your head to the right. Inhale and exhale (for four counts).
6. Return to the center position. You can do this stretch a couple of times or more, or you can do it once to each side and hold the positions longer.

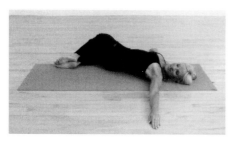

EXERCISE 3

Repeat stretch exercise 1.

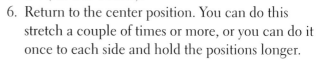

The Fat Flush Fitness Plan

Rest and Renewal: Phase 3

Now that you're in phase 3, you can go back to the kinds of workouts you did before you began the Fat Flush Fitness Plan, as long as you make sure to get five days of cardio, two days of the Lymph-Fit/Compound Strength and Stretching workout, and cool-down stretches after all your exercise sessions. You may find that you're no longer satisfied to lounge around on the weekends, that you need to be moving your muscles and using your body in a vigorous way. Or you may discover that you really treasure your days of rest, that you cherish both your five workout days and your two days off.

Either way, don't forget the three days of aromatherapy baths and the dry-brush and lymphatic massages. You'll find more details on these elements in Chapter 7.

We've designed phase 3 so that you can stay on both the fitness and the eating plans for the rest of your life. Although building in workout time becomes second nature for some women, others continue to struggle with their schedules. So we're including one last set of workout calendars, just to remind you that you'll only keep on this plan for as long as you stay committed to it. The rewards are enormous—but the commitment has to come from you. We hope that by now, it's a commitment that you'll make with eagerness and pleasure, today and every day for the rest of your life.

My Fat Flush Fitness Plan Workout Calendar: Phase 3 (weeks 1 and 2)

	Monday	Tuesday	Wednesday	Thursday	Friday	Saturday	Sunday
8 A.M.							
9 A.M.							
10 A.M.							
11 A.M.							
Noon							
1 P.M.							
2 P.M.							
3 P.M.							
4 P.M.							
5 P.M.							
6 P.M.							
7 P.M.							
8 P.M.							
9 P.M.							
10 P.M.							

My Fat Flush Fitness Plan Workout Calendar: Phase 3 (weeks 3 and 4)

	Monday	Tuesday	Wednesday	Thursday	Friday	Saturday	Sunday
8 A.M.							
9 A.M.							
10 A.M.							
11 A.M.							
Noon							
1 P.M.							
2 P.M.							
3 P.M.							
4 P.M.							
5 P.M.							
6 P.M.							
7 P.M.							
8 P.M.							
9 P.M.							
10 P.M.							

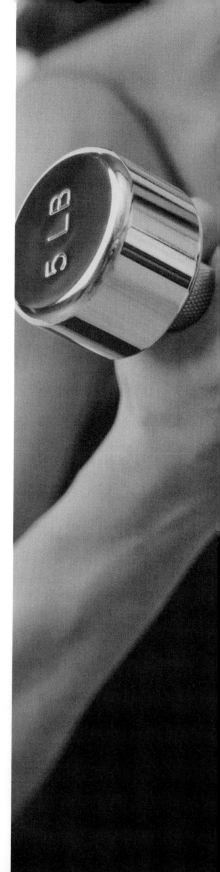

6
Phase 3: Variations

We are wiser than we know.
—Ralph Waldo Emerson

We all know that variety is the spice of life. Would it surprise you to learn that variety not only spices up your exercise plan, but is also a crucial component for its continued effectiveness? If you just follow the same exercise routine, week after week, your muscles get far too comfortable and you might start losing fitness benefits. The idea is to keep moving forward.

In this chapter, we'll give you some options for varying your phase 3 workout—four additional fitness routines that you can feel free to substitute for the Lymph-Fit/Compound Strength and Stretching Workout. You'll keep on doing your cardio, with its warm-up and cool-down stretching, but instead of sticking with the Lymph-Fit/Compound Strength and Stretching Workout, you can choose any of the four variations described in this chapter.

Your goal is to shock the muscles, as we say in the fitness world. Part of our survival as human beings depends on being able to continually meet new challenges, expanding our physical and mental capacity by eternally trying unfamiliar things. Numerous studies have shown that mental signs of aging—forgetfulness, confusion, brain fog—can often be reversed when older people continue to engage in new learning experiences, *demanding that their brains remember new information, master new skills, or take part in new experiences. Your muscles work the same way, you've got to make it just a little bit difficult for them so they'll stay vital, vigorous, and flexible.*

If you are not challenging your muscles, your body will adapt to a routine repeated for too long, and you'll begin to feel the effects of calorie conservation— the dreaded plateau. One way you can tell you've hit a plateau is that you start to feel bored or listless after your workout, rather than energized and inspired.

You can break through plateaus by changing your program every six to eight weeks. You can modify the exercises, the repetitions, the sets, or the routine itself, to keep yourself challenged and to continue the physical transformations for which you are striving. Variety also reduces the likelihood that you'll get bored or find your motivation slumping. You'll have new challenges toward which to work.

So whether you go for lots of variety or prefer more subtle changes, get ready to spice up your exercise life. You'll be amazed at how good it feels.

Recipe for Spicing Up Your Exercise Plan

Each of the four following Fat Flush fitness routines can be used as alternatives to the Lymph-Fit/Compound Strength and Stretching Workout. Each continues to build on the benefits you've already gained, including muscle strength, muscle endurance, muscle tone, and lymphatic stimulation.

- Variation 1: Strength Training Workout Using Dumbbells
- Variation 2: Advanced Strength Training Workout Using Dumbbells
- Variation 3: Intermediate Workout Using Resistance Bands
- Variation 4: Workout Using Stability Ball

Each of these workouts should begin with our old friend the Sun Salutation warm-up and should end with five to ten minutes of cool-down stretches.

Dumbbells

To carry out the Fat Flush Fitness Plan alternative workouts at home, you'll need to invest in several sets of dumbbells. These short, handheld bars with weights at each end are easy to use and need very little storage space (unlike the larger barbells). Dumbbells are used in pairs and come in 1-pound increments. The weights you'll need will depend in part on the size of the weighted ball you used for your Fat Flush Strength Ball workout. If you are using a 6-pound ball, you'll probably start with 5-pound dumbbells. However, we suggest you actually try a set of biceps curls before you buy; you should be able to lift the weight twelve or so times, with the last two reps being a bit difficult but not so hard that you lose your form. We recommend that you purchase at least four pairs of dumbbells, in about 2-pound increments; for example, 5, 8, 10, and 12 pounds for women and 8, 12, 15, and 20 pounds for men. Overloading the muscles will increase your strength. As you gain strength, you will be able to increase the weight of the dumbbells you use.

Varying Your Routine: A Cost-Benefit Analysis

If you DON'T vary your routine . . .

- Your metabolism adapts to your new level of activity, and you stop losing weight—and maybe even start gaining back some weight.

- Your muscle firmness and tone won't improve.

- You'll reach a plateau with your endurance.

If you DO vary your routine . . .
- Your metabolism is continually "challenged" with weight loss/maintenance benefits.

- Your muscles will continue to get stronger and firmer.

- Your endurance will continue to improve.

Variation 1: Strength Training Routine Using Dumbells

	EXERCISE	MUSCLE GROUP	REPS	SET
1	Chair Squat with Weights	quads, gluteals, abs	12–15	1
2	Alternating Lunges	quads, gluteals, hamstrings	10*	1**
3	Standing Calf Raise	gastrocnemius, soleus	15	2
4	One Arm Dumbbell Row	latissimus dorsi	8–12*	2**
5	Bent-Leg Dumbbell Row	latissimus dorsi	8–12	1
6	Dumbbell Chest Press	pectoralis major	8–12	1
7	Dumbbell Shoulder Press	deltoids	8–12	1
8	Alternating Dumbbell Front Shoulder Raise	anterior deltoids	8–12*	1**
9	Alternating Biceps Curl	biceps	12–15*	1**
10	Alternating Hammer Curl	biceps, brachioradialis	12–15*	1**
11	Triceps Kickback	triceps	12–15*	1**
12	Triceps Extension	triceps	15	1–2
13	Oblique Abdominal Crunch	obliques	15	1–2
	Basic Abdominal Crunch	rectus abdominus	15*	1–2
14	Reverse Curl	lower abs	15	1

*Both right and left
**A set consists of an equal number of reps, both right and left

Variation 1: Strength Training Workout Using Dumbbells

EXERCISE 1: CHAIR SQUAT

1. Place a chair behind you and face away from it.
2. Holding a dumbbell in each hand, bend your knees and lower your buttocks until it just barely touches the chair; then come back up (this is one rep). Be sure not to let your knees go any farther forward than your toes. Do the squat by bending at the hips and lowering your buttocks down, rather than by bending forward with your knees jutting out.

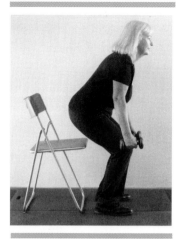

For variety, you may raise your hands and arms up to a position parallel to the floor as you are squatting down, and then drop them back to your sides as you are coming up.

Muscles targeted: lower body (gluteals, abs, and quadriceps)

EXERCISE 2: ALTERNATING LUNGES

1. Stand straight, feet shoulder-width apart, hands on your waist. Step forward with the right leg.
2. Lower yourself down by bending both knees into a lunge position. In this position, your left knee should be an inch or so above the ground. Your right (working) leg should be bent in a right angle, and (very important) your knee should be directly above your ankle, so that your lower leg is perpendicular to the floor. Don't let your right knee go forward past the big toe of your right foot.
3. Raise back up to the starting position (that's one rep).
4. Repeat for the number of reps specified in routine.
5. Reverse the process and start with your left leg coming forward. Repeat for the specified number of reps. (One set for this exercise consists of an equal number of reps for the right and left sides.)

Muscles targeted: lower body (quadriceps, hamstrings, and gluteals)

EXERCISE 3: STANDING CALF RAISE

1. Stand straight and tall, holding a dumbbell in each hand.
2. Raise yourself up on your toes by bringing your heels off the ground.
3. Lower back down (that's one rep).

Muscles targeted: calves (gastrocnemius)

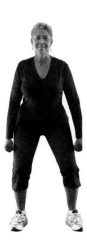

EXERCISE 4: ONE-ARM DUMBBELL ROW

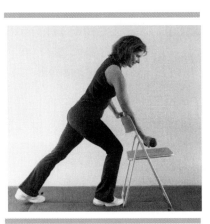

1. Bend over a chair or bench. Rest one hand on the bench and hold a dumbbell in the other, letting it dangle straight down. Make sure your back is straight. (Imagine your back as a tabletop.)
2. Bring the dumbbell up by bending your elbow and lifting it toward the ceiling. Imagine a puppeteer has a string attached to your elbow and is gently drawing it up toward the sky. Stop when the dumbbell reaches your side.
3. Lower your arm back down to the starting position.
4. Repeat for the specified number of reps.

   Muscles targeted: back muscles (latissimus dorsi and rhomboids)

EXERCISE 5: BENT-LEG DUMBBELL ROW

1. Stand with your knees slightly flexed and your body bent forward. Hold a dumbbell in each hand and allow your arms to hang straight down from your shoulders with your palms in (toward your body).
2. Keep your elbows close to your sides as you pull the dumbbells up as high as possible, contracting the muscles in your upper back.
3. Slowly lower the dumbbells back to the starting position.

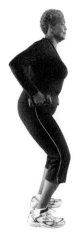

Muscles targeted: back (latissimus dorsi)

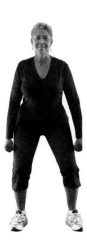

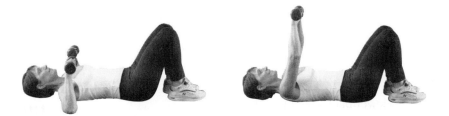

EXERCISE 6: DUMBBELL CHEST PRESS

1. Lie on the floor, knees bent, and feet firmly planted.
2. Take a dumbbell in each hand, palms facing toward your knees, elbows pointed out perpendicular to your body.
3. Your hands should be in line with your mid-chest area.
4. Press the dumbbells straight up toward the ceiling in an extended position, leaving a slight bend in your elbows (do not lock out elbows).
5. Slowly lower dumbbells back to starting position and repeat. That's one rep.

Muscles targeted: chest (pectoralis major)

EXERCISE 7: DUMBBELL SHOULDER PRESS

1. Stand with feet shoulder-width apart, knees slightly flexed (do not lock out knees). Abdominals pulled in.
2. Hold a dumbbell in each hand and bring dumbbells to shoulder level with your palms facing away from your body.
3. With a controlled motion slowly push the dumbbells straight up above your head, keep elbows slightly bent (do not lock out elbows). You should be able to see elbows with your peripheral vision, otherwise your arms are too far back.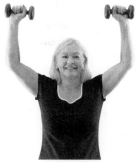
4. In a controlled motion bring dumbbells back down to starting position (that's one rep).

Muscles targeted: shoulders (deltoids)

EXERCISE 8: ALTERNATING DUMBBELL FRONT SHOULDER RAISE

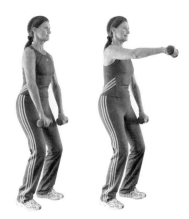

1. Stand with your feet shoulder-width apart, knees slightly flexed. Hold one dumbbell in each hand, arms straight down in front of your thighs, palms facing your body .
2. Slowly raise one arm in front of your body until it is about shoulder level.
3. Slowly lower the dumbbell back to the starting position.
4. Repeat with the other arm, alternating right and left.

Muscles targeted: shoulders (anterior deltoids)

EXERCISE 9: ALTERNATING BICEPS CURLS

1. Stand with a pair of dumbbells in your hands, palms facing out, and your feet shoulder-width apart (6.15).
2. Keeping your elbows stable, raise your right arm toward your right shoulder (6.16).
3. As you bring your right arm down slowly, raise your left arm up to your left shoulder.
4. Bring your left arm down slowly as you lift your right arm toward your right shoulder.
5. Continue alternating right and left arms.

This exercise can also be performed just as effectively by raising (and

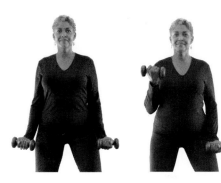

lowering) both arms together. Called a bicep curl in some of our routines, this version can replace alternating biceps curls at any time for variety with no loss of effectiveness.

Muscles targeted: arms (biceps)

EXERCISE 10: ALTERNATING HAMMER CURL

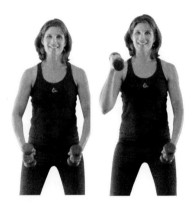

1. Stand with your feet shoulder-width apart, knees slightly flexed. Hold a dumbbell in each hand, arms hanging straight down, palms facing in.
2. With your elbows held at your sides, raise one dumbbell until your forearm is vertical to the floor) and your thumb faces your shoulder.
3. Lower dumbbell to the starting position and repeat with the other arm.

Muscles targeted: arms (biceps, brachioradialis)

EXERCISE 11: TRICEPS KICKBACK

1. Bend over a chair or a bench. Rest one hand on the bench and hold a dumbbell in the other, letting it dangle straight down. Make sure your back is straight (imagine your back as a tabletop).
2. Bring the dumbbell up by lifting your elbow toward the ceiling while bending your elbow as much as possible, thus bringing the dumbbell in toward your shoulder. This is the starting position for the triceps kickback.
3. Keeping your top arm steady, simply extend your arm back all the way until it is in a straight line.
4. Squeeze for a second and then bring the dumbbell back in toward your shoulder to the starting position (that's one rep).

Muscles targeted: arms (triceps)

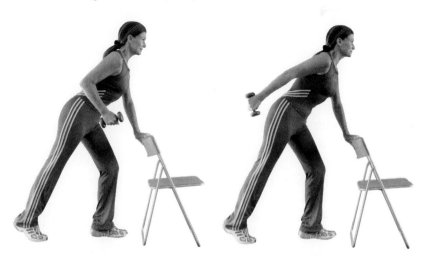

EXERCISE 12: TRICEPS EXTENSION

1. Hold one dumbbell overhead with both hands, standing with knees slightly bent, shoulder-width apart.
2. With your elbows overhead, lower your forearms behind your upper arms by flexing your elbows. Keep your elbows pointed to the ceiling and your upper arms close to your head. (Be careful not to hit the back of your neck with the dumbbell.)
3. Raise the dumbbell overhead by extending your elbows.
4. Repeat for the specified number of reps.

Muscles targeted: arms (triceps)

EXERCISE 13: OBLIQUE ABDOMINAL CRUNCH

1. Lie on the floor with your legs bent, your feet flat on the floor, and your hands clasped behind your head with your elbows touching the ground. Imagine Velcroing your lower back to the floor. This may feel like doing a small pelvic thrust slightly forward. Keep your lower back nice and stable in this position.

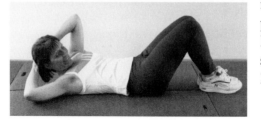

2. Curl up, with a twist to the side; aim your left shoulder toward your right knee.
3. Come back down (not quite to resting position, so you still keep tension on the muscles) and come back up to the other side, this time twisting so that your right shoulder is aimed toward your left knee.
4. Lower back down, remembering not to go all the way to the rest position (that's one rep). (Remember, one rep is a twist to the right and a twist to the left.)

Muscles targeted: Side muscles of the abdominal region (obliques)

You can also do a basic abdominal crunch starting in the same position as in the oblique version. However, instead of curling up side to side, you curl your upper body forward, holding the highest position for a full second.

EXERCISE 14: REVERSE CURL

1. Lie on the floor with your hands at your sides or under your hips.
2. Lift your feet from the floor, knees at a 90-degree angle.
3. Pull in your abdominals and lift your hips in two counts until your buttocks and tailbone are off the floor. Hold for two counts.

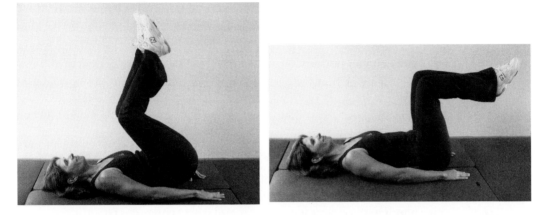

4. Slowly lower back down. Exhale as you lift, inhale as you lower; be sure you keep your upper body on the floor at all times.

Muscles targeted: lower abs

Variation 2: Advanced Strength Training Routine Using Dumbbells

Do the same exercises as in variation 1, but repeat the routine twice.

	EXERCISE
1	**Exercises 1–12** without pausing in between
	Short rest
2	**Repeat Exercises 1–12** without pausing in between
	Short rest
3	**Repeat Exercises 13–14 (Abs)** You may briefly rest between exercises

Variation 3: Intermediate Workout Using Resistance Bands

The following equipment will be used for variation 3.

RESISTANCE BANDS

Resistance bands are another way to strength train. The bands are made of durable rubber and can be purchased with cords or plastic handles attached. The handles make it easier to hold an end in one or both hands, such as when you perform a biceps curl. The handles are impractical, however, for exercises that require you to wrap the band around your foot or hand. Because bands are inexpensive, you should invest in several. Some are flat and wide, while others resemble surgical tubes. In general, the shorter and/or thicker the band, the harder it is to pull and the more resistance it provides. Experiment with different shapes, sizes, and thicknesses to determine which band you like best for each exercise. As you become stronger, you may want to use heavier bands with more resistance. Have all your bands within reach as you begin your workout. The Intermediate Workout Using Resistance Bands employs resistance bands with handles and without handles.

Guidelines for Using Resistance Bands

- Condition of the Band: Check frequently for holes and tears by holding your band up to a light. If you find even the slightest tear, replace the band immediately.
- Standing on the Band: If an exercise calls for you to stand on the band with your feet together, place both feet on the center of the band and then step one foot out to the side so that you have about six inches of band between your feet. This prevents the band from sliding out from under you. Make sure the band is securely in place before each exercise.
- Control Movement: Because of the elasticity of the band, it is important to maintain control of the exercise being performed during both the contraction and extension phase of the movement. If the tension on the band is released abruptly, the band returns to its normal length very quickly and could cause injury.
- Correct Positioning: When performing upper body exercises, stand with your feet shoulder-width apart, buttocks and stomach pulled in, and knees slightly flexed. This position stabilizes the lower back.

EXERCISE 1: RESISTANCE BAND SQUAT

1. Standing, hold handle of resistance band in each hand. Use a band with handles.
2. Place both feet approximately shoulder-width apart in the center of the band (make sure resistance band is secure under your feet).
3. Holding both handles, bring your hands up to shoulder height, palms facing away from your body; keep your hands in this position as you do squat exercise.
4. Keeping your head up, bend your knees in a slow, controlled manner until your thighs are parallel to the floor.
5. Slowly straighten your knees (don't lock out knees) as you stand up back in starting position.
6. Do one set of ten to fifteen reps.

Muscles targeted: lower body

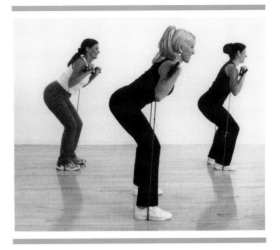

EXERCISE 2: RESISTANCE BAND HIP ABDUCTOR

Use a band with handles.

1. Place both of your feet hip-width apart on the center of the band. Cross the band over so it crosses the body and position your hands so that they are at hip level with elbows slightly bent.
2. Keeping your knees slightly bent, chest up, shoulders down, and abdominals contracted as you abduct your left hip (sidestep with your left leg) as wide as you can.
3. Bring your right leg toward your left leg. Bring it back only to where your feet are still hip-width apart so that there is still resistance.
4. Complete the required repetitions on the left side, and then abduct your right hip (sidestep with your right leg) to complete the set (ten reps with each leg).

Keep your back straight, knees slightly bent, and toes forward throughout the entire exercise.

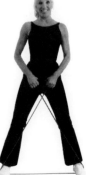

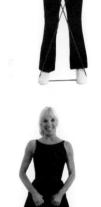

Muscles targeted: gluteals, lower body

EXERCISE 3: UPRIGHT ROW

Use a band with handles.

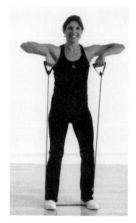

1. Stand with your feet slightly less than hip-width apart and your knees flexed, with the middle of the band under both feet. Hold a handle in each hand with your arms extended toward the floor, palms facing the body.
2. Slowly bend your arms, pulling the band up toward your chest. Your elbows should be pointing to the side. Return to the starting position and repeat (one set equals ten to fifteen reps).

Muscles targeted: upper body

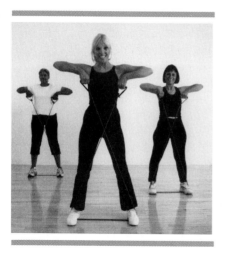

EXERCISE 4: LATERAL RAISE

Use a band with handles.

1. Standing on the band with your feet shoulder-width apart and your knees slightly flexed, hold the handles of the band and cross the band over so it crosses your body. Keep your palms facing your thighs and bend your elbows slightly. Your spine should be in a neutral position.
2. Exhale as you slowly bring your arms out to the side, keeping a slight bend in your elbows, until they reach shoulder level. (In the upper position your hands should not be higher than your elbows or shoulders. Do not shrug your shoulders when you raise your arms.)
3. Slowly return to the start position in a controlled manner (one set is ten reps).

Muscles targeted: deltoids

EXERCISE 5: BICEPS CURL

Use a band with handles. (If you are prone to elbow injuries, use a lighter resistance band, or you might want to skip this exercise.)

1. With a handle in each hand and your palms facing up, stand on top of the center of the band so that your feet are hip-width apart.

Straighten your arms down at your sides. Stand tall with your abdominals pulled in and your knees relaxed.

2. Bend your elbows and curl both arms up until your hands are in front of your shoulders. Don't let your elbows move forward as you curl. The band should be tight at the top of the movement. Slowly straighten your arms. Never lock out your elbows (one set equals ten to fifteen reps).

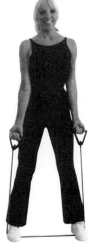

Muscles targeted: biceps

EXERCISE 6: STANDING TRICEPS EXTENSION

Use a band without handles.

1. Standing with good posture, hold the ends of the band in each hand and place the band behind your head with your arms bent at a 90-degree angle.

2. Extend one arm to the side. Return to the starting position and repeat on other side. For more intensity, extend both arms together (right and left counts as one rep; do ten reps).

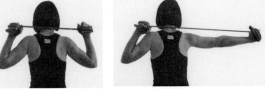

Muscles targeted: triceps

EXERCISE 7: FLOOR CHEST FLYES

Use a band without handles.

1. Lie face up with your legs bent and feet on the floor. Place the band under your midback and wrap the ends of the band around each hand.

2. Straighten your arms to your sides with your upper arms on the floor and your elbows (slightly bent) in line with your shoulders. Extend your arms over your chest, bringing your hands together. Release and repeat (do ten to fifteen reps).

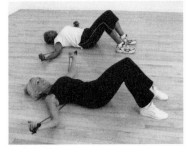

Muscles targeted: chest

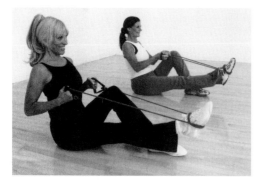

EXERCISE 8: CALF PRESS
Use a band with handles.
The calf press targets your calf muscles. It also strengthens your shins, upper back, and biceps, especially if you keep tension on the band as your toes move both toward and away from you.

1. Holding one end of the band in each hand at waist level, sit on the floor with your right leg straight out in front of you and left knee bent. Wrap the band around the ball of your right foot. Bend your right knee slightly and lift it up in the air. Sit up straight and don't round your back.

2. Point your toe as you pull back on the band. Hold this position a moment and, while maintaining your pull on the band, flex your foot and pull your toes back as far as you can. Complete the set and then do the exercise with your left foot (your right knee should be bent). Do five reps with each leg.

Muscles targeted: calves, shins, upper back, biceps

EXERCISE 9: HAMSTRING STRETCH
Use a band with handles.

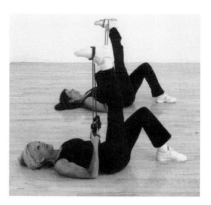

1. Lie face up with your legs straight. Bend your right leg and wrap the band around the ball of the your right foot. (Bend the left knee.)

2. Extend your right leg toward the ceiling, heel up. Hold the handles in both hands and keep them close to your shoulders. Release and repeat on the left side (do one rep on each side, holding one minute).

Muscles targeted: lower body

When you have finished your resistance band workout, do the abdominal exercises that follow.

	EXERCISE	MUSCLE GROUP	REPS	SET
1	**Oblique Abdominal Crunch**	rectus abdominus	15	1–2
	Basic Abdominal Crunch	obliques	15	1–2
2	**Reverse Curl**	lower abdominal muscles	15	1

Variation 4: Workout Using Stability Ball

The following equipment will be used for variation 4.

Stability Ball

Stability ball training has long been used in rehabilitation. Today, not only do medical doctors, osteopathic specialists, chiropractors, physical therapists, and other fitness professionals use the ball to treat and rehabilitate physical injuries, along with mainstream practitioners and the public, they are also getting "on the ball" and using it to prevent more serious physical problems before they occur.

The benefits of stability ball training come from maintaining proper alignment on the ball, which stimulates the body's natural motor reflexes and encourages the body to react as a whole. It's actually the *instability* of the support that challenges the entire body, since when using the ball correctly, the body is required to utilize various muscles for stabilization. These muscles may not have been previously challenged using traditional, well-supported exercise positions. Stability balls challenge core strength by putting to work the core muscles in the body (the muscles located deep in your pelvis, abdomen, trunk, and back), which are essential for good posture, spinal alignment and support, balance, and all movement, both for everyday activities as well as exercise.

As you work out on the ball, you will find that it is especially effective in targeting your abdominal and lower back muscles. Even while training other muscle groups, the abs and back are working to balance and stabilize the body. The ball is ideal for stretching and offers additional alternatives to traditional static stretching.

Stability balls come in a variety of sizes. The best way to figure out the right stability ball for you is to sit on it. Your hips and knees should align at about a 90-degree angle. The chart that follows will help you choose the best size.

Stability Ball Sizes

YOUR HEIGHT	BALL HEIGHT	BALL SIZE
Up to 4' 10"	18 inches	Small
4' 10" to 5' 5"	22 inches	Medium
5' 6" to 6' 0"	26 inches	Large
6' 0" to 6' 5"	30 inches	Extra large
Over 6' 5"	33 inches	Extra, extra large

Instructions and Guidelines for Using the Stability Ball

Keep the following in mind when exercising using a stability ball:

- Perform all exercises slowly and deliberately.
- Follow the exercise descriptions carefully.
- Work into a movement gradually so that you get used to the pattern of the exercise and learn how to balance your body properly.
- If at any time you feel discomfort or pain, stop immediately and check your form. Severe discomfort should never accompany any exercise program.

Before starting to exercise or stretch with the stability ball, you should become comfortable with it by finding your neutral lumbar spine position.

- Slouch slightly while on the ball by rounding the lower and upper back.
- Begin bouncing lightly (an added bonus: bouncing stimulates lymph flow).
- Let your body automatically find your straightened posture, which will allow you to maintain your balance and continue bouncing. The straightened posture, which occurs when you bounce up, is your neutral lumbar spine position.

When your bounce feels comfortable, you've found your center of gravity, and even shifting it slightly will require you to correct it to stay on the ball. This simple exercise will challenge your core muscles and introduce you to the stability ball before you move on to variation 4.

We would like to point out just a few precautions for using the stability ball. If you often experience unexplained loss of balance (such as sudden blood pressure changes potentially leading to light-headedness or dizziness), you should avoid using an exercise ball, since balance is so important when using it. You should always exercise with the stability ball on a soft floor (avoid concrete or tile, for example) in order to avoid injury if you should fall off.

EXERCISE 1: SEATED CORE WARM-UP
1. Sit with good posture on the stability ball, hands on your hips (6.41).
2. Tilt hips side to side, then back to neutral position. For variation, tilt hips forward and back or in a circular motion (do ten to twelve reps; right and left counts as one rep; forward and back counts as one rep.)

Muscles targeted: lower body

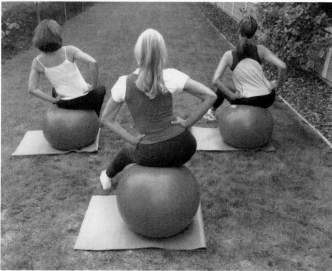

EXERCISE 2: SEATED BALANCE
1. Sit on the stability ball with your hands on your hips, as you did in exercise 1.
2. Keeping your abdominals contracted, lift your left foot off the floor. Release. Repeat on the other side. (Do ten to twelve reps; right and left counts as one rep.)

Muscles targeted: balance, core stabilization

EXERCISE 3: PUSH-UPS ON STABILITY BALL

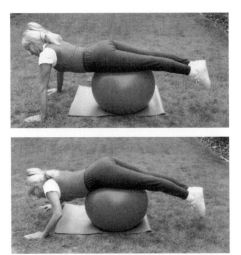

1. In a face-down position, place your thighs and pelvis on the stability ball and your palms on the floor, with your hands aligned under your shoulders.
2. Lower your chest toward the floor, keeping your upper arms and elbows close to your rib cage as you bend your arms. Release and repeat. (Do ten to twelve reps.)

Muscles targeted: chest, shoulders

EXERCISE 4: LATERAL FLEXION

1. Lie on your side with the stability ball under your waist and hips. Extend your legs and put one foot in front of the other. Bend your arms and place your hands by your ears.

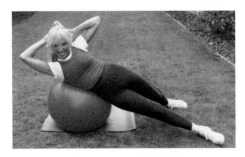

2. Drape yourself over the ball, then lift your torso in the opposite direction, bringing the side of your rib cage to the side of your hips. Don't let your pelvis roll forward or back on the ball. Return to the starting position and repeat. Do the right and left sides (ten reps each side).

Muscles targeted: core muscles, abs, back

EXERCISE 5: ABDOMINAL CRUNCH

1. Lie face up with the stability ball under your hips, midback, and lumbar spine.
2. With feet on the floor, bend your legs to 90 degrees and align your knees over your ankles. Cross your arms over your

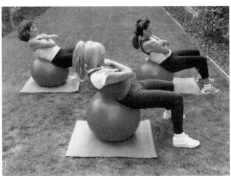

chest, bringing your hands to the opposite shoulder.
3. Move your rib cage to your pelvis as you curl your upper body forward. Your lumbar spine and hips should remain touching the ball. Release and repeat (for ten to twelve reps).

(The difference between doing a ball crunch and a crunch on the floor is that the ball crunch forces you to maintain your balance while you perform the exercise, targeting the abdominal and back muscles more directly.)

Muscles targeted: core muscles, abs, back

EXERCISE 6: OBLIQUE CURLS

1. Lie face up with the stability ball under your hips, low back, and midback. With your feet on the floor, bend your legs to 90-degrees and align your knees over your ankles (Figure 6.51).
2. With your arms bent, place your hands by your ears. Curl up to your right side. Your lumbar spine and hips should remain touching the ball (Figure 6.52). Release and repeat on other side. (Do ten to twelve reps; right and left count as one rep.)

Muscles targeted: obliques

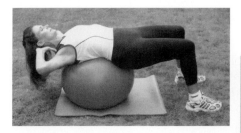

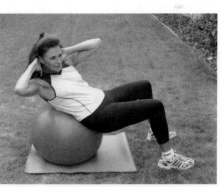

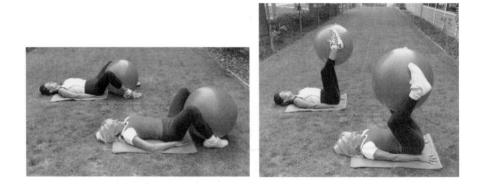

EXERCISE 7: REVERSE ABDOMINAL CURL

1. Lie face up with your hands between your low back and the mat. Bend your legs to 90 degrees and hold the stability ball between your feet.
2. With control, lift your tailbone off the mat and bring your pelvis toward your rib cage. Release and repeat. (Do ten to twelve reps.)

Muscles targeted: core muscles, abs, back

EXERCISE 8: LUMBAR ROLL

1. Lie face up with your legs bent at a 90-degree angle and the stability ball under your legs (the ball should be touching your calves, hamstrings, and glutes). Extend your arms out on the floor at shoulder height, palms up.
2. Without letting your shoulders lift off the ground, slowly roll the ball to the left side, and then reverse the movement to the right. (Do ten to twelve reps; right and left counts as one rep.)

Muscles targeted: core muscles, abs, back

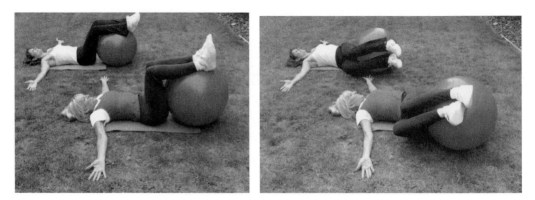

Stretches for the Stability Ball, Variation 4

STABILITY BALL STRETCH 1: SUPINE HIP STRETCH

1. Lie face up with the right leg extended, your calf resting on the ball. Bend your left leg and cross it over the extended right leg, placing your left ankle just above the right knee.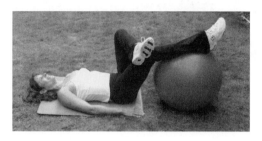
2. Bend the right leg 90 degrees, pulling the ball toward you. Place your left hand on the left knee without pulling on your knee. Hold and repeat on other side (hold thirty seconds or more on each side).

Muscles targeted: hamstrings, lower back

STABILITY BALL STRETCH 2: ABDOMINAL STRETCH

1. Begin with your head and shoulder blades on the stability ball in a supine position, with your knees directly over the top of your ankles .
2. Inhale slowly; extend back on the ball, raising your arms over your head. Hold for one minute.

Muscles targeted: core muscles, abs, back

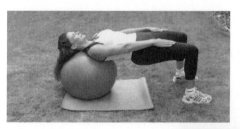

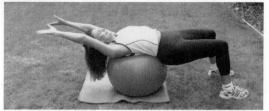

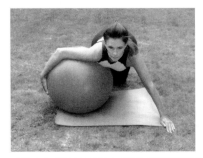

STABILITY BALL STRETCH 3: KNEELING CHEST STRETCH

1. Kneel on your hands and knees with the ball on your right side. Extend your right arm and place it across the top of the stability ball. Maintain a neutral spine position
2. Gently lower your chest toward the floor without straining your shoulder. For variation, roll the ball slightly forward or back to change the angle of the stretch. Hold and repeat on other side. Hold for thirty seconds or more on each side.

Muscles targeted: chest

STABILITY BALL STRETCH 4: LOW BACK STRETCH

1. Lie face down on the stability ball.
2. Position the ball under your abdominal area and allow your arms and legs to drape over the ball and relax toward the floor. Hold one minute or more. Stretches the back.

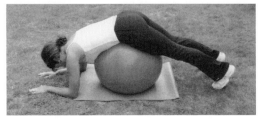

STABILITY BALL STRETCH 5: KNEELING SHOULDER STRETCH

1. Kneel behind the stability ball with your arms straight and palms together.
2. Roll the right triceps and elbow on the ball with your right shoulder pointing to the floor and your left shoulder to the ceiling. Your fingertips should point away from the ball. Release and repeat on other side. Hold for thirty seconds or more on each side.

Muscles targeted: shoulders

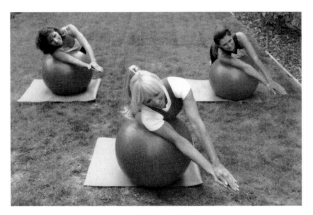

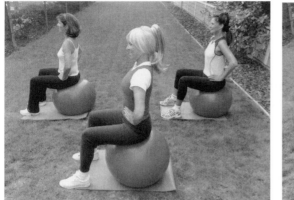
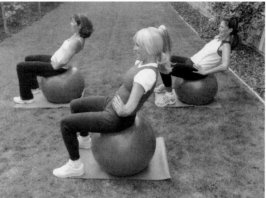

STABILITY BALL STRETCH 6: LUMBAR MOBILITY STRETCH

1. Sit on the stability ball with your legs bent and knees over your ankles. Place your hands on your hips.
2. With control, use the abdominals to move the pelvis forward and backward. Imagine rolling your tailbone toward the front of the ball, then toward the back of the ball. Repeat four times for twenty to thirty seconds.

Muscles targeted: lower back

STABILITY BALL STRETCH 7: SEATED NECK STRETCH

1. Sit in a neutral position on the stability ball with your shoulders relaxed.
2. Place your right palm on your right thigh and your left hand on the side of ball, with your fingertips pointing to the floor.
3. Tilt your head to the right, allowing your right ear to move to the right shoulder. Then slowly tilt your chin away from the right ear and toward the ceiling. Release and repeat on other side. Take your time and move slowly.

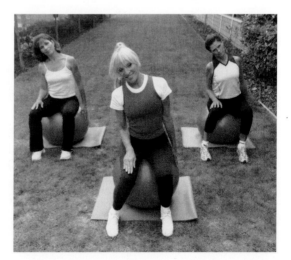

Muscles targeted: neck, upper back

How to Vary Your Routine

It's easy to vary an exercise routine once you know how. First, of course, there's the obvious way, just switch to a whole new routine. Do one of the four routines included in this chapter.

But you can also play around with the Lymph-Fit/Compound: Strength and Stretching Workout or with one of the variations in this chapter, or you can change one of the following elements:

- duration (how long your routine lasts)
- frequency (how often you do it)
- intensity (how hard you're working)

Let's say, for example, that you're doing the dumbbell workout with lighter weights, two times a week. In four weeks, you might vary your *intensity*, choosing a heavier set of weights. Then, four weeks later, vary your *frequency* to three times a week.

Vary Your Strength Routine

- Switch equipment: vary among the strength ball, dumbbells, and resistance bands.
- Go for a heavier strength ball or heavier weights.
- Practice lifting more slowly for a more challenging workout.
- Vary the exercises you do with your strength ball or weights.
- Find new exercise combinations and patterns, including varying the order in which you do the exercises.

Staying Motivated: Defining Your Goals

Mei was worried. She'd lost the weight she wanted, and she'd enjoyed the workouts on the Fat Flush Fitness Plan. She'd reorganized her kitchen, bought the *Fat Flush Cookbook*, and warned her family that this new diet was now her way of life. "And I feel so good eating this way, that I'm sure I'll keep going," she told us. "What I'm not so sure about is my fitness routine. I just get so busy. I'm not a very disciplined person. How do I stay active?"

Joanie asked Mei why she wanted to stay active.

"Oh," Mei replied quickly, "I know it's better for my health . . . and I'll have more energy . . . and . . ."

"No," Joanie said. "Why do you want to stay active? Why is it important to *you*?"

Mei thought a minute. "You know what I keep thinking?" she finally said. "Before, when the weekend came around, I barely had enough energy to chauffeur the kids from one play date to the next. But this past few weeks I actually *felt* like taking them to the park and, of all things, flying a kite with them. And the day they were off on a class trip, do you know what I did? I actually spent the afternoon walking around downtown, looking at the photo galleries. It sounds stupid, but with three kids, if I get a day to myself, I usually just want to crawl into bed and take a nap. This was the first time in a long time that I wanted to be out in the world, doing things."

Mei had connected to her reasons for staying active, and suddenly, she was far more confident about remaining motivated. Joanie suggested that she make herself a little reminder of her motives—Post-it stuck on her mirror, saying "Kite and Galleries," or maybe a piece of the kite's tail wound around her bed-post, to keep her personal goals front and center. "In the end, you're the only one who *really* knows why you want to exercise," Joanie told her. "Doing it for someone else won't work. Just keep asking yourself why you care, and you'll realize that you always have your own personal answer to that question."

To help you identify your own objectives, here's a list of some of the goals we have heard over the years:

- To keep the weight off.
- To keep my energy levels up.
- To have more patience with my kids.
- My sex life has really improved, and I want to keep it that way!
- I like the clothes I can fit into now.
- I plan on living to a ripe old age. When I'm eighty, I want to be traveling, going to the movies, taking walks on the beach, just like I do now.
- I've always dreamed of climbing mountains, and maybe now I can.

Being aware of your own fitness goals is always the most important thing you can do to keep yourself motivated. Now, what are *your* fitness goals? Take a few minutes to jot them down in your journal, or, if you prefer, fill out this questionnaire:

1. Now that I've been exercising for a while, some changes I've noticed are

_____

_____

_____

_____

_____

_____

2. Some changes I'd still like to see in the next twelve weeks are

_____

_____

_____

_____

3. When I think about where I'd like to be next year, I envision

_____

_____

_____

_____

4. Staying fit would help me achieve that goal because

_____

_____

_____

_____

5. When I think about where I'd like to be in five years, I envision

_____

_____

6. Staying fit would help me achieve that goal because

_____

_____

_____

_____

7. When I think about my lifelong dreams, I envision

_____

_____

_____

_____

_____

8. When I think about staying fit for the rest of my life, I envision

_____

_____

_____

_____

9. When I think about *not* staying fit, I imagine

_____

_____

_____

_____

10. In order to stay fit, I'm willing to

_____

_____

11. To demonstrate my commitment to myself, I will take this one specific action:

_____

_____

_____

_____

_____

Staying Motivated: Keeping Yourself on Track

There's no question about it: defining your goals is the most powerful fitness motivator there is. But even when you keep the big picture in mind, it's helpful to give yourself small boosts along the way. Here are some more tips for staying motivated as you continue to exercise:

- Stay proactive. The only way to get something done, especially if you're a busy, active person, is to commit to it. That means putting your workout on your schedule every day, planning your week with exercise in mind, and taking your appointment with exercise as seriously as you would any other appointment. If you tell yourself that you'll get to the doctor when you think of it, you never will, but if you have a 3 o'clock appointment, chances are you'll show up. Find ways to make your exercise dates as unbreakable as any other kind.
- Combine exercise with other things you like to do, or other things you have to do. Be creative. Take the dog out, or walk to the store instead of driving, or get off the bus one stop early on your way to work. Find ways to build exercise into your day so that it becomes a normal part of your routine.
- Treat yourself. Do you like listening to books on tape, or to a particular type of music? Maybe you can make your exercise time an opportunity for some pleasant listening. Or, if you're a museum fan, could you bribe yourself with a walk to the museum? Imagine how much fun it will be to look at the art when you're glowing with the health and vitality of a brisk walk!

- Measure your progress. Some people find that a pedometer, heart rate monitor, or stop watch makes a terrific motivational tool. Knowing how far you've gone, how fast you've gone, or how fit you are can inspire you to keep coming back for more, especially if you record your daily progress in your fitness journal.
- Join a team. When you know that your teammates are relying on you, it's hard to let them down. Staying fit becomes part of the web of your relationships, with motivation coming from your teammates as well as yourself.
- Take advantage of your competitive spirit. If you're the type who likes to win, enter a contest or participate in an athletic event. Find a way to connect your exercise to another goal that you already care about.
- Connect to Mother Nature. If you find it inspiring to walk in the woods, hike up a mountain, or experience the great outdoors from the back of a horse, use these natural treats as powerful motivators. The goal is to figure out what excites you and then use it to move you toward fitness.

And a Few More Tips . . .

- Rebounding is great for the lymphatic system, so try to get some in if you possibly can, even if it's just five minutes a day. You can always combine five minutes of rebounding with other types of cardio.
- It's better to work out five minutes than not to work out at all. So if a day comes when you've got no time, find five minutes. Excuse yourself from the meeting and walk briskly around the block. Or do some stretches in your kitchen. At the very least, do some deep breathing. Even if you work out only five minutes a day for a whole week, you're benefiting more than if you were totally sedentary. And having stayed active will make it that much easier to get back into a longer workout when you're ready to resume your program.
- Figure out a good mental script for yourself, with answers for all your favorite self-sabotaging excuses. If you find yourself thinking, *I really don't have time*, answer yourself firmly, *Then I'll just take five minutes*. If you tell yourself, *I'm really too tired*, you might answer, *Remember how good you'll feel as you're stepping out of the shower*. Having clear physical memories of your peak exercise experiences helps, too!

The Fat Flush Fitness Lifestyle

Remember: *You* are the creator of your own lifestyle. The choices you make determine who you are. If you devote part of your day to healthful exercise, that's who you are. If you spend the entire day sitting on the couch, that's who you are. You have the power to create yourself, every single day. And if you don't take hold of that power, well, that's a choice, too.

What's exciting about the Fat Flush fitness and eating lifestyles is that they really will sustain you for life, supporting your body, mind, and spirit so that you are free to create the life you want. Congratulations. Now you have everything you need to stay fit the rest of your life!

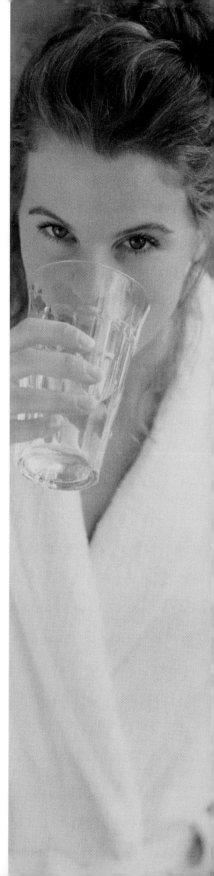

7

Taking Care of Yourself: Massages, Bathing, and Sleep

You only live once, but if you work it right, once is enough.
—JOE E. LEWIS

Marcy was the type of superorganized person who planned her entire day, right down to the two and a half minutes she needed to remove her makeup before bed. She had taken to the Fat Flush Fitness Plan like a duck to water—except for the baths. Committed as she was, she just couldn't see the point of wasting twenty minutes luxuriating in a tub when she could finish a shower in five minutes.

Yasmin was the first to admit she was "a real space queen." "Somehow," she told us, "the day just gets away from me." She had always started her day with an early-morning yoga session, so it wasn't hard for her to add the rest of the Fat Flush Fitness Plan to that session. But committing to massages and baths seemed more than she could manage. "I know why exercise is important," she said. "But aren't these other things optional? I mean, they're nice and all—but if I've got time when the day is over, I'd rather watch TV."

When Alex learned that the Fat Flush eating and fitness plans called for her to get eight hours of sleep each night, she told us bluntly, "Well, I get six hours of sleep during the week, and I'm not interested in changing that part of my life. I need the time to get things done, and I don't see what difference it makes. I make up my extra sleep on the weekend."

If you you still question why we want you to bathe, get massaged, and log eight hours of sleep each night, you can see that you're not alone! When we started the Fat Flush Fitness Plan, we thought the hardest part would be convincing women to get regular exercise. Imagine our surprise when it turned out to be a lot more difficult to persuade them to take it easy!

As the stories we've just quoted make clear, there are usually three major issues that get in the way of women taking care of themselves:

1. "I don't have time." If we feel too busy, it can be hard to make the time for any part of a new routine. . . .
2. "They're just extras." . . . and since we are too busy, what do we get rid of first? The extras, naturally! It just makes sense . . .
3. "I don't really need them." . . . especially since we didn't need them anyway!

There's just one problem with this way of thinking. You actually do need the baths, massages, and sleep time—just as much as the workout. So this chapter is dedicated to the reasons you need these elements of our plan, and to help you find the time, commitment, and energy to build them into your life.

If you already love the idea of sleep, massages, and long, fragrant baths? Read on anyway—the time may come when you'll have to convince someone else *about why these apparent luxuries are crucial for your health.*

Lymph-Friendly Massage

In Chapter 1 we told you that the lymphatic system doesn't have a pump. That means you need to move the lymph through its channels some other way. An active lifestyle, including the Fat Flush Fitness workouts, is a terrific start. But it's also helpful to get regular massage.

Massage helps your lymph move through its channels and nodes more efficiently, nourishing your tissues and making white blood cells—the mainstay of your immune system—available to your entire body. Massage also stimulates your circulation, freeing toxins and waste products and carrying them down into the lymph system which then removes them from your body.

Therefore, massage can be a potent form of healing. A study from the University of Miami found that massage actually increased the number of natural killer cells in the immune system, boosting your ability to resist disease.[1] The technique also helps release endorphins so you feel less pain and muscle soreness—especially important when you take up a new routine or activity.

Massage also reduces stress, which, as discussed, is a key factor in weight gain and weight retention. Remember that stress leads to high levels of cortisol, a powerful hormone that helps your body retain fat, especially in the abdominal region. So anything that lowers cortisol levels is a huge help in your diet and fitness efforts. Cortisol may also help promote the development of cellulite, especially around your abdomen. (For more on cellulite, see Chapter 8.)

Meanwhile, by stimulating your circulatory system, massage improves the flow of oxygen and nutrients to every cell, boosting your energy levels and helping to create healthy, glowing skin. Massage also promotes regular sleep, which reduces stress, lowers cortisol levels, and so, indirectly, can lead to weight loss.

Phases 1 and 3: The Full-Body Fat Flush Lymphatic Massage

The full-body Fat Flush lymphatic massage—part of phases 1 and 3 of the Fat Flush Fitness Plan—is unlike any type of massage you're familiar with. Unlike the tissue- and muscle-based massage you may have had at a spa or salon, lymphatic massage focuses on manual lymphatic drainage—stimulating your lymphatic system to drain lymph more efficiently. So while you're enjoying the relaxing, soothing experience of being massaged or massaging yourself, you can take further comfort in the knowledge that this procedure can actually increase the volume of your lymph flow by as much as twenty times.

Over 70 percent of your lymph vessels are located just beneath the skin, and they're very delicate—only one cell thick. So the Fat Flush lymphatic massage is a very gentle technique, designed to prevent damage to these tiny channels.

Many professional massage therapists are trained in manual lymphatic drainage. You can also find a friend, lover, or family member to massage you, or follow our guide for self-massage.

The Full-Body Fat Flush Lymphatic Massage—Thirty Minutes, Once a Week

We think you'll enjoy this massage so much that you'll look forward to your once-a-week date. But to boost your motivation, remind yourself that this procedure is only effective when you do it regularly. So during phases 1 and 3,

Finding a Massage Therapist

- Ask friends, family members, and coworkers for referrals. You'll be surprised to find how many people are getting regular massages these days!

- Ask at your local gym, health club, or YMCA. Many of these organizations have professional massage therapists on staff. Some YMCAs even offer courses in massage.

- Check your local telephone directory—"massage," "spa," "salon," and "bodywork" are good key words.

- Visit the Web site of the American Massage Therapy Association, which offers a free service to connect clients with its members. (See Chapter 10 for more information.)

Note: Although many reputable bodyworkers aren't licensed or certified, you're looking for a specialized type of massage, so you probably need someone who is highly trained. About thirty states and the District of Columbia license massage therapists. A massage therapist can also become certified by the National Certification Board for Therapeutic Massage & Bodywork, which requires five-hundred hours of classroom instruction from an accredited school, a written examination, and continuing education each year. Be sure to ask any therapists you find whether they are qualified to perform manual lymphatic drainage. If they haven't heard of it, they're not qualified!

make sure your weekly calendar includes at least one half-hour massage date.

You'll want to find a warm, quiet area where you're not likely to be interrupted. A chilly temperature will make it hard to relax, as will the prospect of an imminent knock on the door or a visit from your toddler. Maybe you can tempt your husband with the prospect of a massage for him when you get done with yours!

Lie on the floor, sit on a chair, or lie on your bed if your mattress is firm—whichever is more comfortable. The direct contact between your hands and your skin is very healing, so wear as little clothing as you can—another reason to find a warm and private place!

You might want to have some massage oil or lotion ready, just to make it easier to rub your hands over your skin. Whether or not you use body oil, you should always apply a moisturizer to your face before a massage. Massaging dry facial skin causes unnecessary pulling and stretching.

Lymph flows toward two major vessels in your chest, so the direction of your massage should be in the same direction; that is, toward your heart. Be sure to massage both the left and right sides of your body. And always begin with your face and neck. Thirty percent of your lymph nodes are located below your jaw.

STEP 1: LYMPHATIC FACIAL MASSAGE

Ann Louise first learned this basic part of the massage from skin care specialist and veteran Fat Flusher Karie Wagner on our charter Fat Flush cruise. Ann Louise liked it so much, she adapted it for the program.

1. Using the side of your index fingers, briskly massage up and down on your forehead. Using the side of your index fingers, briskly massage the sides of your face, from the temples near the hairline to the bottom of your ears.

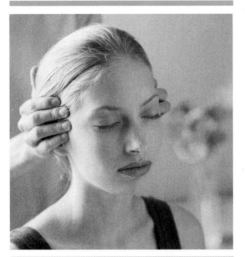

2. Using the sides of your index fingers, start at your cheekbone beside your nose. Hook your finger under the cheekbone and gently vibrate your fingers back and forth. Gradually move down the cheekbone, vibrating your fingers, until you reach the center of the cheekbone, directly below the center of your eye. Using the same vibrating motion, finish this region by placing the underside of your thumbs under the cheekbone directly below the outer corner of your eyes and moving toward the center of the cheekbone.

3. Open your mouth slightly to create slackness in the hollow directly below your cheekbone. Using the tips of three fingers, massage both sides in a circular motion. Place your thumbs, underside against your skin, behind your jawline and just below your ears. Vibrate your thumbs and move down the jawline until your thumbs meet at your chin.

4. Bend your head to the left so your neck muscles are relaxed on the left side. Hold the four fingers of your right hand straight and firmly together. Start just under the jawline on the left side and slide your

right hand down your neck and across your shoulder. Repeat ten times on the left side, then carry out the same process on the right side. You may feel a tingling sensation in your neck and arm as the lymph flows.

STEP 2: UPPER BODY LYMPHATIC MASSAGE
Once you have the lymph flowing in your face and neck, move down to your arms and torso. Remember to move your hands toward your heart.

1. Begin on your right arm at the wrist. Using the fingers of your left hand, smooth and stroke the inside of your arm from the wrist to the inner elbow. Use light, feathery strokes. When you reach the elbow, gently massage with a circular motion, then continue the light stroking movement along the inside of your upper arm. At the armpit, use your thumb and fingers to gently squeeze the skin, forcing the lymph out. Use light, feathery strokes from the armpit across the right breast toward the center of your chest. This moves the lymph to the two major blood vessels in the chest, along which it flows to the kidneys and liver for elimination. Repeat this process on the left side.
2. Rub in a gentle circular motion between the breasts. Tenderness in this area indicates you may have some lymph congestion; the tenderness will disappear once you've done the massage several times and cleared the congestion.
3. Starting about an inch below your breasts, gently stroke your skin outward and upward toward your armpits. Continue across your rib cage, working from the center outward and upward until you reach your waist.

STEP 3: LOWER BODY LYMPHATIC MASSAGE
When you get to your lower body, your massage strokes move upward, toward your heart.

1. Start with your right leg. Use one or both hands to massage the base of each toe and between each toe with circular motions. Then stroke from the toes toward the ankle, using a feathery motion. Massage in a circular motion all around the ankle. Stroke upward along the calf until you reach the knee. Use both hands to massage around the

entire knee with circular motions; don't forget the back of the knee, where several lymph nodes are located. Stroke along your thigh using your fingertips or the palms of your hands. At the back of your thigh, use a circular motion to massage at the base of the buttock, an area particularly prone to lymph stagnation. Continue your stroking motion in toward the crease at your groin, where many lymph nodes are located. Repeat this process on the left side.

2. In the groin area, work both sides at the same time. Stroke upward and diagonally across the groin with the flat of your hand on each side. Move your hands toward each other, so they come together over your abdomen. Repeat this process as often as you need to in order to cover the entire groin area.

3. From your waist, stroke both sides downward over your abdomen toward the groin.

This full-body massage will take about thirty minutes. You may feel some discomfort after the first few sessions as you feel your lymph flow increasing and as more waste is carried out of your body. Some women feel temporarily bloated and swollen from the renewed flow, while others have minor reactions to the toxins. Think of this discomfort as analogous to the temporary aches and pains you feel in your muscles as you're using them for the first time. Once your system is working as it should—muscles engaged, lymph flowing—you'll feel terrific!

A Quick Alternative: The Fat Flush Pump Massage—Five Minutes

Although we strongly encourage you to find thirty minutes for the Fat Flush full-body massage, we know you're busy—so for those weeks when life sabotages all your well-laid plans, here's a quickie alternative. In just a few minutes, you'll get lymph flowing from head to toe. You will need a partner to perform this massage for you, though, so start building up your favor bank. You'll be glad you did!

For the Lymph Pump massage, lie flat on your back on a mat or carpeted floor, with your feet bare. Wear loose, light clothing—or, if you're comfortable, no clothing at all. Here are the directions to relay to your massage partner:

1. Rest one hand, palm up, under my leg just above my left ankle, cradling my Achilles tendon.

2. Place your other hand on the bottom of my foot with the palm resting against the ball of my foot and your fingers curled over my toes.
3. Push on the ball of my foot so that it makes a 90-degree angle with the floor.
4. Pull back on my toes until the ball of my foot is as close to the floor as possible.
5. Repeat this pumping action ten times, making sure my entire body moves with each push and pull. Then repeat with my right foot.

Going with the Flow

Some people feel light-headed when they stand up after a massage, especially if they're not used to this form of treatment. The feeling can result from the release of toxins, which will soon pass out of your body through urine or sweat. Or, you may be reacting to the increased amount of blood now circulating throughout your system. If this is a concern, have a glass of water ready so you can sip it slowly before getting up.

Although most people don't get sore muscles from our gentle lymph massages, this does occur occasionally. Do some stretches, take a hot bath with Epsom salts, and drink a few glasses of water to help the soreness pass.

Phases 2 and 3: Fat Flush Dry-Brush Massage

Another technique to stimulate lymphatic flow is dry-brush massage, or skin brushing. Dry-brush massage promotes lymph flow and blood circulation, stimulates oil-producing glands in your skin and helps enhance your immune system. This simple technique also helps lessen the appearance of cellulite; rebuilds new, strong connective tissue; and promotes toned, supple skin, especially as you lose weight.

Your skin is the largest organ of your body, and dry-brushing is one of the best things you can do for it. Your skin is designed to help rid your body of wastes as you perspire. Dry-brushing will remove dead layers of skin, open the pores, and remove toxins, leaving a youthful, healthy glow.

To get started, find a good brush at your local bath and beauty store, health food store, or department store. Look for a medium-firm brush with natural bristles—nylon or other synthetic bristles tend to be sharp and might damage your skin. Select a brush at least as large as the palm of your hand, with a long handle to reach your back.

Keep your brush clean by washing it frequently in warm, soapy water. Make sure it air dries completely before you use it again. Once a week, soak your brush for thirty minutes in a solution of one quart water and a few drops of Clorox bleach or tea tree oil (a natural disinfectant).

In case you were wondering why we waited until phase 2 to introduce the Fat Flush dry-brush massage, it's because most people who start the Fat Flush Plan have weakened connective tissues from years of sluggish lymph flow and accumulated toxins. Dry-brushing this damaged tissue can cause bruising and discomfort. By phase 2, though, your connective tissues should be stronger and more resilient, and dry-brushing will be very therapeutic.

You can dry-brush yourself at any time, but we don't advise waiting until the last few minutes before bedtime, as the brushing tends to have a stimulating effect that might interfere with sleep. If you dry-brush first thing in the morning, you'll feel energized all day. You'll probably want to shower or bathe after brushing, to wash away the dead skin.

The Fat Flush Dry Brush Massage—Five Minutes, Two Times a Week

Feel free to work your way up to five times a week. Your skin will thank you for it, and so will your lymphatic system.

1. Open the primary lymphatic ducts by gently finger-massaging just below your collarbone and on the left and right groin areas. This only takes a few seconds.
2. Begin the brush massage with the soles of your feet. Brush vigorously in a circular motion. How firmly you press depends on how toned and healthy your skin is. As your skin becomes healthier, you will be able to apply more pressure, create better circulation, and bring increased energy into the skin. Using short, upward strokes, gradually move over your feet and legs. Continue brushing upward over your stomach to your breasts and over your buttocks to your waist.
3. Repeat the circular motion on the palms of your hands and then use short, upward strokes on your hands and arms. Brush down from your neck out to your shoulders and down to your breasts and down your back. As with other massage techniques, always stroke toward your heart.

Don't brush skin that's irritated or bruised. And avoid brushing your face—the skin is too sensitive there.

Soaking Up the Power of Aromatherapy

Despite Marcy's skepticism about making time to soak in the tub, an aromatherapy bath can actually be a potent way to support both the Fat Flush eating plan and the Fat Flush Fitness Plan. Bathing reduces stress, eases aching muscles, opens your pores, gives your skin a healthful glow, and stimulates your lymph flow by pulling toxins and wastes from your body through perspiration. Taking a hot bath before bed will help you sleep—a crucial part of fitness and weight loss as well.

Aromatherapy can supplement the power of bathing if you add the right essential oils to your bathwater. Essential oils are distilled from the roots, leaves, and flowers of wild or organically grown plants. When you rub them on your skin or put them in your bath, they are quickly absorbed by both your skin and your nose, carrying their subtle messages to your limbic system—the portion of your brain that creates a sense of wellness and harmony. From there, they travel to your hypothalamus, the gland that regulates anxiety, depression, and hormonal balance.

Essential oils have been credited with numerous effects, including:

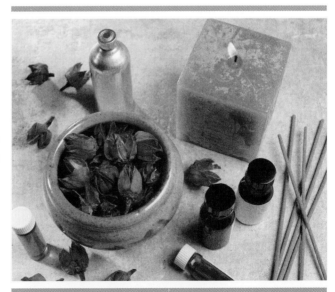

- reducing water retention and fat deposits
- alleviating stress and anxiety— which reduces cortisol, which in turn aids weight loss
- reducing muscle soreness

Studies have also shown that certain essential oils can stimulate the hypothalamus to:

- suppress your appetite. Alan Hirsch, M.D., director of the Smell and Taste Research Foundation in Chicago, has shown peppermint activates the portion of the hypothalamus that regulates our sense of fullness.[2]

- relieve pain. Studies in England and elsewhere have noted the powerful effect of lavender and rose oils to overcome intense pain. Through the hypothalamus, their scents inspire the thalamus gland to produce encephalin, a natural painkiller and antidepressant.[3]
- stimulate your immune and lymph systems. Lemon and other oils trigger the release of noradrenaline, which both fights fatigue and boosts your immune and lymph systems.[4]

Plus, let's face it—they just smell good! The pungent scent of cinnamon, the spicy aroma of bergamot, the zesty smells of lemon and orange stimulate your senses and reawaken your awareness of your physical self. There are many utilitarian reasons to lose weight and become fit—combating heart disease, lengthening your life span, boosting your energy levels. But it's nice to remember that the ultimate purpose of these plans is to enable you to enjoy your life, take pleasure in your body, and renew your spirit.

So open up to aromatherapy by putting some essential oils into your warm bath, enabling the oils to penetrate your skin.[5] Choose two or more oils from the Lymph-Friendly Essential Oils list, and add a total of ten drops into the flowing water as you fill your tub. (Don't overdo it—these are potent substances and using them to excess could produce an allergic reaction or other unwelcome side effects.) Then soak for twenty minutes—at the end of the afternoon, to help you release workday stress and transition to a relaxing evening, or an hour or so before bedtime to help you sleep.

What You Must Know About Using and Caring for Essential Oils

- Avoid oils that contain synthetic ingredients, which might produce an allergic reaction. Buy only 100 percent pure and natural oils. (Check out Chapter 10 for some ideas on where to buy your essential oils.)
- Store the undiluted oil tightly closed in a blue or amber glass bottle, away from the sunlight or heat—your refrigerator is an ideal spot.
- Avoid using your essential oils near candles or open flames; they're highly flammable!

- Never swallow these highly concentrated oils, and keep them away from your eyes, ears, and mucous membranes. Don't apply them directly to your skin—use a carrier oil. And keep them away from children and pets.
- Use only the recommended amount of oil. These substances are potent, so don't "overdose!"

If you're pregnant or nursing, do not use any essential oils without consulting your doctor.

Tubs Versus Toxins

Aromatherapy baths aren't the only way to turn your bathtub into a therapeutic refuge. Ann Louise's mentor, alternative medicine pioneer Dr. Hazel Parcells, provided this therapeutic bath formula for Joseph Dispenza's *Live Better Longer*;[6] her theory is that it helps build your immunity by raising the acid level of your body at the cellular level. The higher acid level creates an environment in which bacteria and viruses do not flourish. The bath will help your detox process, and you can also use it to combat the onset of a cold or flu.

1. Fill the tub with hot water—95 to 100 degrees Fahrenheit—and add two cups of apple cider vinegar.
2. Soak in the tub until the water is cool.

Lymph-Friendly Essential Oils

Here are some oils recommended for their ability to decongest the lymphatic system.[6]

- Clary sage—supports endocrine function and helps to release fluid from swollen tissues.

- Cypress—strengthens weak connective tissue, restores skin tone, enhances circulation, releases toxins.

- Grapefruit—dissolves fatty deposits, with toning and tightening qualities. It is also highly antimicrobial.

- Juniper—promotes the elimination of toxic waste and helps to reduce fluid retention.

- Lemon—disssolves fatty deposits, as the other citrus oils do, while also purifying the system.

- Lemongrass—tones and strengthens connective tissue and stimulates lymphatic drainage; also acts as a diuretic to purge excess fluids from the system.

- Orange—stimulates circulation and helps to increase lymphatic flow, relieving puffiness and water retention.

- Rose and lavender—reduces stress and controls cravings.

- Rosemary, lavender, peppermint, and mandarin orange—reduces pain from muscle ache, headache, or arthritis.

3. As you soak, sip a glass of warm water that contains one tablespoonful of apple cider vinegar.
4. Wait at least four hours before showering.

Here's my bathing formula to combat jet lag:

1. Dissolve 2 pounds of sea salt or rock salt and 2 pounds of baking soda in a tub of water as hot as you can stand.
2. Soak in the tub until the water is cool.
3. Wait at least four hours before showering.

Sleep: The Secret Fitness Aid

Lack of sleep can make you fat. Remember, cortisol is one of the hormones that stimulates fat storage and revs up your appetite to make sure you have energy for all the stressful challenges that you face. When you are sleep deprived, however, your body interprets this as a stressor—after all, it takes a lot of extra energy to go without sleep—so your cortisol levels remain elevated, and so does your appetite for carbohydrates.[7]

Other kinds of hormonal problems can be triggered by lack of sleep. For example, a study at the University of Chicago found that young adults who were sleep deprived showed a significant loss in their ability to process glucose (blood sugar), which caused their bodies to produce more insulin.[8]

Insulin is the key hormone that controls our blood sugar levels after we consume carbohydrates. Insulin metabolizes blood sugar so that muscle tissue can use it for fuel. It also helps store excess blood sugar in the liver and tissues as glycogen, or in our bodies as fat. So excess production of insulin can result in too much blood sugar being stored as fat, interfering with weight loss efforts. This is why the Fat Flush Plan's balanced diet of lean protein, low-glycemic carbohydrates, and "good" omega-3s and omega-6s is so important. It helps keeps our insulin levels low. Fat-deprived people eating too many carbohydrates—even complex carbohydrates—program their insulin levels to remain high. The insulin, in turn, instructs their bodies to store fat.

Excess insulin also triggers a whole host of symptoms, including irritability, difficulties with memory and concentration, and food cravings. Too much insulin production can also exhaust the islet of Langerhans—the part of your pancreas that produces insulin—which can put you at risk for diabetes.

Levels of the hormone leptin also drop when you don't get enough sleep. Leptin helps regulate carbohydrate metabolism, so lack of sleep can boost your carb cravings.

You also need deep sleep to produce growth hormone, which helps give you supple skin.[9] Growth hormone also causes your body to burn fat in order to repair the tiny tears in your muscles caused by exercise. This gives your body a higher muscle to fat ratio, which boosts your metabolism, helping you to lose weight and keep it off.

Growth hormone is released while you sleep, raising gradually from about 10 P.M., and peaking at about 2 A.M. Eating a light, low-carb Fat Flush "friendly" snack—a fruit smoothie or a deviled egg—just before you retire can boost growth hormone production even more.

Although everybody's needs are different, most people require eight hours of sleep each night. You may already have noticed that the Fat Flush eating and fitness plans will actually help you fall asleep more easily and sleep more deeply. But if you have any trouble falling asleep or staying asleep, here are some suggestions that might help:

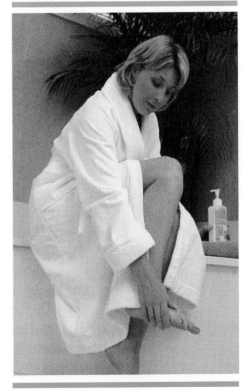

- Create a ritual around sleep. Doing a few things that signal your body to prepare for bed can help you feel drowsy at the appropriate time. Avoid overly stimulating TV or music; don't take on any work or family problems close to bedtime; and by all means, avoid sweets, carbs, alcohol, and caffeine before bed—they are all real sleep disturbers! (We know you're avoiding them anyway, but make a special point of avoiding them in the late evening.)
- Finish your exercise at least two hours before bedtime. Exercise alerts your body to rev up— you want to slow down. Even if a workout makes you tired, it also wakes you up, so work out no later than two hours before your bedtime for maximum sleep support.
- Try a hot bath. According to the National Sleep Foundation, taking a fifteen-minute hot bath ninety minutes before going to bed brings on sleep more quickly.[10] Many other studies have

found that a bath inspires frequent episodes of deep sleep.[11] A warm, scented bath can be a terrific part of your bedtime ritual, especially after a stressful day.

- Eat lightly before bedtime. You get home late from work or after your child's Little League practice and you're famished. Unfortunately, your body works hard to digest a heavy meal—and that can interfere with restful sleep. If you must eat within three hours of going to sleep, try a Fat Flush "friendly" light stir-fry or veggie omelet to keep both hunger pangs and heartburn from disturbing your sleep.

- Restrict your bed to sleeping, sex, and—if you must—some light bedtime reading. Don't work, watch TV, or do any other stimulating activity in bed. (Even if you find TV relaxing, its flickering electronic signal actual stimulates your brain and keeps you up.) School your body to respond to a consistent signal: bed is for winding down; somewhere else is for revving up.

- Make your bedroom a sleep sanctuary. Buy a comfortable mattress, sleep on clean sheets, and keep your room cool—60 to 65 degrees. Use light-blocking shades or lined drapes to keep out light. Control noise with earplugs, double-paned windows, heavy curtains, or "white noise" from a fan or air purifier. Use a humidifier if the room is too dry.

- If you can't fall asleep within fifteen minutes, get up. Do something you enjoy, to avoid the sense that you're punishing yourself for staying awake. Read something light, listen to soothing music, or take a hot bath or shower. Relax with deep breathing or meditation—or, if a problem is plaguing you, take steps to solve it if you can, or to consciously release it until tomorrow if you can't. You might write briefly about the problem, along with an "appointment" the next day to work on a solution. Then put the paper aside and try going back to bed.

- Avoid taking a nap after 4 P.M. or sleeping for more than one hour during the daytime. If you're sleeping during the day, and you have no problem sleeping at night, then don't worry about it; your body knows what it needs. But if you're in a cycle of naps and insomnia, do your best to resist napping. Your body needs help in resetting its clock, and natural tiredness is part of that assistance.

- Maintain your waking and sleeping times even on weekends. It's important to understand that you don't really "catch up" with extra sleep on the weekend. Your weight retention, carb cravings, and hormonal imbalances affect you during the week no matter how well you sleep on Saturday and Sunday. And if you're cranky, tired, or depressed during the week, you've already paid a high price for your sleep deficit, no matter how well you sleep on the weekend.

Poor Sleep May Signal a Health Problem

If you're not sleeping well, you might have hypothyroidism, sleep apnea, or some other disorder that requires special treatment. So talk to your physician or a sleep specialist if you're plagued with any of these symptoms:

- Loud snoring
- Chronic exhaustion
- Sleep apnea (interruption of breathing for several seconds; your bed-mate will often spot this problem before you do)
- Restless leg syndrome (an unpleasant sensation in your calf that makes you feel that you must move your legs)
- Chronic irritability
- Difficulty falling asleep within thirty minutes of going to bed
- Difficulty returning to sleep after awakening during the night or early morning

A Total Approach to Health and Weight Loss

We live in a culture that promotes the idea of pushing ourselves to the limit—at work as well as at play. Sadly, we often confuse the healthy self-challenge that is central to any good diet and fitness program with a type of overexertion that not only damages its benefits but also sabotages our weight loss efforts.

Too often, our confusion is supported by our friends, families, and coworkers. People who will gladly help us make time for taking a half-hour run are far less sympathetic to our need for a half-hour bath. Family members who readily understand our need to cut back on carbs may be slow to understand why we need to boost our intake of sleep.

As with everything else in this plan, we believe that knowledge is the key to power. Now that you know how central sleep, massage, and bathing are to your health, weight loss, and overall well-being, we hope you'll feel empowered to add these crucial elements to your life. Even if—like Marcy, Yasmin, and Alex—you find it difficult to take the plunge, we challenge you to give this approach a try for just thirty days. We're willing to bet that at the end of just one month of this type of self-care, you'll find yourself so energized, serene, and productive that you can't even imagine going back to your old way of life. So take our challenge!

Soak in a tub, take a massage, and get some sleep. It's a great way to feel good—and helps you lose a few pounds.

8
Flush Away
Your Cellulite

*It were not best that we should all think alike, it is
a difference of opinion that makes great horse races.*

— MARK TWAIN

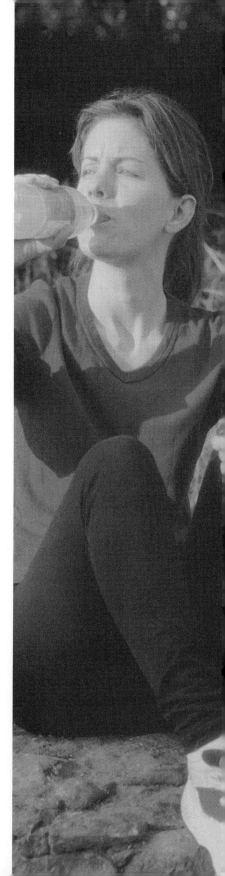

You've lost those stubborn inches. You've gained a tremendous
amount of energy. You have healthy, glowing skin, your eyes have new
sparkle, and your posture is so excellent everyone thinks you're a dancer.
Your friends think you look fabulous, and you feel renewed. There's only
one thing about your appearance that may still concern you—cellulite.

Cellulite is the dimpling of the surface skin of your thighs, buttocks,
and abdomen caused by damage to the fatty tissue that lies just
beneath your skin. Although women of all ages and body types have
cellulite, it's more common in older and heavier women. It's basically
a cosmetic issue—nothing to worry about healthwise. But for many of
us, it's an annoying aspect of getting older and we'd dearly love to be
rid of it.

Although no one is really sure what causes cellulite, scientists have
come up with lots of theories, including heredity, water retention,
excess estrogen, and poor circulation. Some researchers simply dis-
miss it as another type of body fat. We, however, focus on a different

factor—lazy lymphatic and circulatory systems that encourage your body to hold onto its toxins.

There are a few factors that conspire in this process. First, the body tends to store toxins in fat. And women's long-term fat-storage reserves are in the thighs; the lower body has the ability to stockpile six times more fat than the cells in the upper body.

Second, the connective tissue in the female leg forms a fibrous, honeycomb-like pattern in which fat tends to lodge. So fat accumulates in our legs more readily than in our arms.

Third, the legs have a more concentrated network of lymphatic vessels than does any other area of the body. Put these three factors together, and they spell cellulite.

Researchers have also suggested that gaining fat while losing muscle contributes to the appearance of cellulite. Unless you stay on the Fat Flush Fitness Plan—or another strength-training program—you're likely to lose 5 pounds of lean muscle for each decade of your adult life. In those areas where we have the most fat to begin with—the hips, buttocks, and thighs—losing muscle mass means the area has a weaker underlying foundation, causing the fatty tissue to lose its shapeliness. The underlying muscle layer thins as the fat chambers thicken. And the skin, lacking a firm foundation, assumes the irregular appearance of the subcutaneous layer. The result is those telltale lumps, bumps, and "orange-peel" skin that we know as cellulite.

But there's good news on the horizon. The massage, dry-brushing, and bathing that we recommended in Chapter 7 are gentle, but powerful, anticellulite techniques. The aromatherapy massage we'll describe in this chapter also helps reduce the appearance of cellulite, even if technically the fat deposits are still there. And of course, your whole Fat Flush eating and fitness program will boost your sluggish lymphatic system, build up lean muscle mass, reduce fat, and end water retention, as well as help you balance your estrogen levels, thus eliminating many of the factors that cause cellulite in the first place.

How do we know? *Fat Flushers throughout the country have told us that simply by following the diet and fitness plans, they noticed that their cellulite seemed to disappear. Indeed, many women have nicknamed it "the anti-cellulite diet."*

Certainly, many components of *the Fat Flush eating and fitness plan—including the pure unsweetened cranberry juice and water, rebounding, strength training, and massage—combine to give your skin a smooth, toned appearance. And although conventional thinking holds that you can't make cellulite disappear, we've come to believe that these components significantly influence the appearance of cellulite, if not eliminate it altogether.*

So if you'd like to reduce or eliminate the appearance of cellulite, read on. You'll be delighted to find that you're already doing many of the things that will help it to go away.

Identifying Cellulite

Here's the bad news: even if you can't see any dimpling or roughness on your skin, you might still have cellulite. To find out, gently pinch a fold of skin on your upper thigh, the part of the body where cellulite most commonly appears. If you've got it, your skin will have a quilted or dimpled appearance when you pinch it.

Cellulite progresses over time, so the "pinch test" is only the first sign of what you might expect:

Stage 0—No signs of dimpling or bulging when you sit, stand, or pinch. In this case, you don't have cellulite—but the activities outlined in this chapter may help you to prevent it.

Stage 1—Dimpling when you pinch your skin, but not when you sit or stand. You may also see tiny broken veins, feel tenderness when you pinch gently, or bruise easily. At this point, the cellulite has just begun to form. Rigorous application of the techniques in this chapter may enable you to prevent the further appearance of cellulite.

Stage 2—No signs when you lie down, but dimpling occurs when you stand. Your skin may feel cold to the touch, and you may see large broken veins. You won't be able to do anything about the broken veins, but you may be able to reverse some of the dimpling.

Stage 3—Dimpled, quilted skin in all positions. You may feel "islands" of hot skin among areas of cold tissue. Even though your cellulite is far advanced, you'll be able to do quite a bit to flush the fatty deposits out of your skin and restore a healthy, glowing look to your epidermis (the top layer of skin).

Even if you're in top physical shape, with firm, hard muscles, you can still have cellulite, but in that case, it's more likely to be solid or hard. You won't be able to pinch your skin, but you may notice that skin in the affected area is dry or rough. Soft cellulite has a liquid feel as you squeeze it, and the surrounding skin tends to hang more loosely. It also tends to spread over a wider area than the hard cellulite that feels firm.

Whichever type of cellulite you have, however, you'll benefit from cleansing your lymph system and improving your muscle-fat ratio. So take heart. The first step is for you to learn a bit more about what cellulite is and how it is formed.

The Causes of Cellulite

European researchers have generally taken cellulite far more seriously than their American counterparts, using ultrasound, lymphangiography (an examination of the lymph channels), and other sophisticated techniques to studying cellulite. Thanks to their efforts, we now know that cellulite occurs when the fatty tissue just beneath your skin is damaged.

It helps to picture your skin as a series of layers. On top is the epidermis—that's the layer you see. Just under the epidermis is the dermis, also known as the corium. Then comes the upper layer of subcutaneous tissue, which in women contains large oblong fat-cell chambers, separated by connective fibers that are attached to the dermis at one end and the lower layer of subcutaneous tissue at the other end.

As you age, these connective fibers become thinner and less rigid. A number of other factors can weaken them as well: accumulated toxins caused by a sluggish lymphatic system and an overstressed liver; excess fat deposits caused by a deficient diet and lack of exercise; and poor circulation, which leads to a slowdown in venous blood flow.

According to British physician Dr. Elizabeth Dancey, this sluggish blood flow allows toxic wastes to accumulate and blood pressure to build, which in turn weakens the veins' walls.[1] Blood leaks out into the surrounding tissue, your veins don't do their usual efficient job of carrying waste away from your tissues, and the excess waste damages the connective fibers that hold together the various layers of your skin. (As a result, the same factors that create cellulite also seem to lead the development of varicose veins, and the anticellulite tools in this chapter may likewise work to mitigate varicose veins.)

At the same time, a sluggish lymph system is also contributing to the buildup of waste in your tissue. Dancey describes a study at Brussels University using lymphangiograms to examine lymph flow in women visiting a cellulite clinic that found that every woman who had cellulite had poor lymph flow.[2] In the words of Dr. Dancey, "the problem of a deficient lymphatic system must be addressed if cellulite is to be dealt with effectively."[3]

Meanwhile, in the subcutaneous layer just beneath your skin, fat is accumulating within the cells, due again to poor diet and lack of exercise. This accumulation distends the fat cells, enlarging them and causing them to protrude upward. In response to the pressure, the dermis loosens and becomes thinner, and fat cells—which were never meant to leave your subcutaneous layer—migrate on up to the dermis. So the fat cells have ballooned up in size and they're also moving up closer to the surface of the skin; hence, the bumpy appearance of cellulite.

By now you may be wondering why men don't also get cellulite. The answer lies in their tissue structure. Their dermis is thicker than women's, helping it to resist invading fat cells. And their subcutaneous layer contains smaller fat chambers that are themselves crisscrossed by connective fibers. As a result, men's skin is naturally firmer and better toned than women's.

As you can see, we're back to the same matters with which we started: a buildup of toxins in the body and a sluggish lymphatic system, combined with a sedentary lifestyle, stress, fluid retention, and a diet high in processed foods, refined carbohydrates, and saturated fats. These are the factors that create cellulite—and these are precisely the factors that the Fat Flush eating and fitness programs are designed to address. If you follow these plans, your cellulite will look markedly better—and some women have even found that it has completely disappeared.

Overcoming Cellulite: Your Anticellulite Toolkit

Remember, it took years to accumulate your cellulite, so you may need a bit of patience as you work to overcome it. But with this set of anticellulite tools, you've got a fighting chance to achieve clear, smooth skin:

- The Fat Flush eating plan
- The Fat Flush Fitness Plan
- Gels and creams
- Dietary supplements
- Dry-brush massage

Tool #1: The Fat Flush Eating Plan

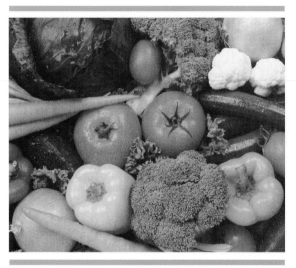

The effectiveness of the Fat Flush eating plan in making cellulite seem to disappear stems from both what it includes and what it avoids. The plan's unsweetened cranberry juice–water mixture and Long Life Cocktail of cranberry juice, water, and psyllium or flaxseed are potent sources of phytonutrients—the special nutrients found in brightly colored fruits and vegetables, including proanthocyanidins and phenols.[4]

Proanthocyanidins strengthen connective tissue by blocking the destructive activity of certain enzymes. They also protect blood vessel walls from damage by free radicals, thought to contribute to cellulite and varicose veins. In addition, they make your capillaries stronger and increase muscle tone in your veins, both of which may help prevent varicose veins. Phenols protect against atherosclerosis and reduce the risk of heart disease, cancer, and stroke.

Cranberries help defeat cellulite in another way as well. Recent research has found that cellulite contains more water-attracting molecules than smooth skin, which may lead to increased water retention.[5] The phytonutrients in unsweetened cranberry juice—and in many other brightly colored fruits and vegetables—have been shown to reduce fluid buildup in tissues.[6]

The Fat Flush eating plan is also based on an understanding that while some fats are bad for our health, other "good" fats are crucial to it. One of those crucial good fats is conjugated linoleic acid (CLA), a dietary supplement that you take daily during phase 3 of the Fat Flush diet. We now know that CLA has the ability to help your body flush out the fat, based on studies like the one headed by Michael Pariza, M.D., who concluded that CLA reduces the body's ability to store fat and promotes the use of stored fat for energy.[7] CLA's impact seems to be especially profound on deeper abdominal fat, suggesting that it might be effective on the fat that gives rise to cellulite as well.

At the same time, the Fat Flush eating plan steers you away from substances that might ultimately promote cellulite. On this plan, you'll avoid caffeine, which can raise blood sugar, insulin, and cortisol, high levels of which ultimately encourage your body to store fat. You'll also avoid high-glycemic carbohydrates and simple sugars, which also encourage fat storage, as well as processed foods, which can overload your body with toxins and promote stored fat.

Tool #2: The Fat Flush Fitness Plan

Thanks to the way rebounding stimulates your lymphatic system, helping to drain waste products and fluids from your tissues, many Fat Flushers begin to see their cellulite diminish soon after starting on the plan. Then, with the introduction of strength training in phase 2, anticellulite efforts get a real boost. Strength training ensures that you will add muscle mass as you lose fat, which, as we've seen, works against the appearance of cellulite. Studies by Wayne Westcott, Ph.D., research director at the South Shore YMCA in Quincy, Massachusetts, confirm the anticellulite effects of building up lean muscle mass. In one study, Westcott found that fully 70 percent of the participants reported they had "a lot less cellulite" after completing an exercise program that included strength training, while the other 30 percent reported having "less cellulite." In other words, 100 percent of the people he studied found that exercise helped reduce their cellulite.[8]

Of course, the Fat Flush fitness program has even more anticellulite effects than most exercise routines because of our focus on cleansing the lymphatic system and promoting lymph flow. Although we didn't actually design the Fat Flush eating and fitness programs to target cellulite, we might as well have!

Tool #3: Gels and Creams

Let's be very clear about this: simply rubbing a beautifully packaged fragrant cream or gel on your thighs will not make your cellulite magically disappear. However, some products have been shown to reduce fluid accumulation, stimulate the release of fatty acids into the bloodstream, and give your skin a smooth appearance.

Gels are water-based, whereas creams are an emulsion of oil and water. Women with oily skin may prefer gels, but be aware that creams contain both oil-soluble and water-soluble ingredients, while gels can carry only water-soluble substances. You can buy anticellulite products online, in health and beauty stores, or in health food outlets. Look for gels and creams that contain the following types of ingredients:

- Centella asiatica (gotu kola)—to improve circulation, strengthen and tone blood vessels, and stimulate tissue repair, including the connective tissue in the subcutaneous layer of the skin.
- Hedera helix (ivy)—to improve fluid drainage in the tissues.
- Cola vera—a natural source of caffeine that stimulates fat cell receptors to release fatty acids into the bloodstream when applied topically. Look for salves with 0.5 to 1.5 percent cola vera extract. (Of course, no matter how much caffeine you rub on your skin, please don't drink any! This potent substance causes small blood vessels to constrict, which actually encourages development of cellulite and varicose veins.)
- Horse chestnut—which contains an active ingredient, escin, that reduces tissue swelling, improves circulation, and has an anti-inflammatory effect. Look for salves with 0.5 to 1.5 percent escin.
- Algae or seaweed, including kelp, fucus, and bladderwrack—to promote firmness of the epidermis and blood circulation in the tissues.
- Silicium—an organic form of silica derived from the horsetail plant that stimulates fat-cell receptors to release fatty acids into the bloodstream, preventing damage to the small blood vessels and ensuring a good blood supply to the skin and other tissues.
- Retinols—to smooth the surface of your skin, minimizing the orange-peel look of cellulite, according to research at the University Medical Center of Liege, Belgium, and elsewhere.[9] The effect apparently comes from the demonstrated ability of retinols to stimulate collagen production, thus strengthening the subcutaneous layer and tightening the skin. Be aware that many people are very sensitive to retinols. Check with your dermatologist before using them.

Tool #4: Fat Flush Anticellulite Supplements

Remember, there's no miracle cure, so you can't get rid of cellulite simply by taking a pill. But escin, the active ingredient in horse chestnut, has been shown to inhibit vein swelling and tone blood vessels, lessening the appearance of varicose veins as well as that of cellulite.

In addition, look for formulas that contain a number of lipotropic elements to help prevent excess fat buildup and thin or emulsify fat for easy movement through your bloodstream (see Chapter 10). Some of these lipotropic elements include

- methionine, an amino acid
- lipase, a fat-digesting enzyme
- phosphatidylcholine and inositol, B-complex vitamins
- L-carnitine, which carries fat to the mitochondria, the "fat furnaces" in your cells that convert fat to energy
- turmeric, dandelion root, milk thistle, and Oregon grape root, which are all lipotropic herbs

A Word of Caution

Herbal supplements may be natural, but they are also a potent form of medication. Why would you take them if they weren't? So be sure to check with a doctor before starting any course of herbal treatment, especially if you're pregnant, nursing, or taking prescription medications. DO NOT take anticellulite supplements if you're on blood-thinning medication. And never take more than the recommended dosage, any more than you would overdose on penicillin or painkillers. Treat herbal supplements with the same caution that you'd use with any other type of medication.

Tool #5: Dry-Brush Massage

We've already explained in Chapter 7 how to do dry-brush massage and why this form of massage is good for your lymph system. Isn't it nice to know that it's good for cellulite, too?

Again, there are no miracle cures! But the circular brushing of your hips, buttocks, and thighs stimulates the movement of your blood and lymph, helping to move these fluids through any circulation-starved areas so they can carry away excess water, toxins, and waste products. It also removes any dead cells that may be clogging your pores, which improves the health and appearance of your skin. Finally, the brushing stimulates your nerve endings, which both improves muscle tone and enhances your immune system.

Creating a New You

You'll notice lots of differences in your appearance after only a few weeks on the Fat Flush fitness and eating plans. Your posture, skin, shape, and tone will all improve dramatically—whether or not you notice an improvement in your cellulite as well. Indeed, these other factors, plus the loss of water weight, false fat, and bloat, will improve the appearance of your skin and shape, even if your cellulite itself remains unchanged.

But if you're like most women we've known, engaging in the Fat Flush fitness and eating plans will affect the appearance of your cellulite—perhaps even quite a dramatic difference. The prospect is certainly an added incentive to clear your system of toxins and flush away the fat!

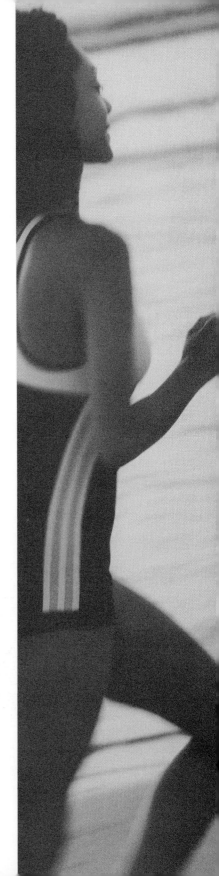

9
Making Fitness Part of Your Life

To fill the hour, that is true happiness.
—RALPH WALDO EMERSON

Kim liked the Fat Flush plans so much, she got all her friends to try the eating plan, and she sent two of her coworkers to enroll in Joanie's fit camps. Yet, she told us a few months after she'd completed the initial twelve weeks of the plan, that she was feeling a bit frustrated. Her job at a media consulting firm required her to take frequent business trips that involved long flights, days jam-packed with meetings, and a total disruption of her schedule. "It's not just the travel, although that's bad enough," Kim told us. "But when I get home, it's really hard to get back into the old routine. I love my rebounder—but on the weeks when I travel, I barely have a chance to use it, let alone do any strength training."

Nikki, too, was enthusiastic about changing the way she ate and bringing the healthful benefits of fitness into her life. But from the moment she started on the Fat Flush eating and fitness plans, she encountered obstacles. One week, her husband's folks were visiting, and between cooking their favorite dishes and showing them around town, Nikki had trouble sticking to the plan's guidelines, let alone finding time to work out. The next week, there was a big birthday celebration for Nikki's sister that took up the entire Sunday that Nikki had set aside for a vigorous day of exercise, an aromatherapy soak, and a massage. The week after that, Nikki's daughter had a minor accident in an after-school soccer game—nothing serious, but it did require a visit to the emergency room and a "cheer-up" trip to the local fast-food place afterwards. "It just seems like something is always getting in the way," Nikki told us, "no matter how hard I try."

You've certainly noticed it yourself by now. You plan a healthy Fat Flush lunch—and then your coworkers convince you to join them at a restaurant where you can't find anything healthy to eat, or where you're just too tempted by the special of the day to remember your diet. You set aside a precious hour for rebounding and a luxurious soak in the tub—and your son comes home with a daunting homework assignment that requires an entire evening of parental assistance. You stick to your plans at home—but can't make them work while you're on a business trip, or on vacation. Or you get tripped up by the holidays, or out-of-town guests, or family obligations, or any one of the thousand and one things that make up our busy lives these days.

Well, guess what? That's never going to change—and thank heavens! Having a full life crammed with unexpected events, family demands, and work-related challenges is a tribute to who you are and the choices you've made. If those choices aren't working for you, then by all means make some changes. But if your only problem is sticking to the Fat Flush plans, then stop worrying. The whole point of these plans is to enrich your life, not to saddle you with more obligations. There are plenty of ways you can work healthy eating and invigorating exercise into your life. All it takes is a little flexibility, some creative planning, and the wish to be kind to yourself. If you begin by saying "What's wrong with me that I can't make this work?" then of course you'll have a terrible time, whether you stick to your Fat Flush plans or not. But if your starting point is to view these plans as tools for you, to make your life happier, healthier, and more satisfying, then take a deep breath, relax, and replace that scolding voice inside your head with one that praises you for your resourcefulness, your rich, full life, and your commitment to yourself. Not only will you feel a whole lot better, you'll be much more likely to make healthier, more satisfying choices.

Visualization: Your Secret Weapon

The first step in incorporating the Fat Flush plans into your life, under any and all circumstances, is to use the powerful tool of visualization. To visualize something is to see it in your mind's eye, as though it were actually happening.

Visualizing can serve two purposes. First, when you visualize yourself in a new situation—arriving in a strange hotel on a business trip, for example—you can better anticipate the obstacles that might arise to keeping up with your fitness routine and plan ahead for how to overcome them.

Second, the mere fact of visualizing—seeing yourself going for a brisk walk in the new city, for example, or imagining yourself taking fifteen minutes to go up and down the hotel stairs for a quick cardio workout—makes it more likely that you'll actually do what you've imagined. Visualizing an activity creates pathways in your brain that are virtually identical to the pathways that are created when you actually perform the action. And we all know how powerful habit can be! If you visualize yourself incorporating exercise on a business trip, for example, it's as though you've already made a habit of doing so.

Use the sample situations on the next page to help you visualize, using a calm moment and the powers of your imagination to come up with creative ways that you can do your work, have your fun, see your friends—and still stick to your Fat Flush plans. We've included some suggestions for what you might imagine, but don't stick to our ideas. Once you put yourself in the driver's seat, you're sure to come up with creative solutions of your own.

Taking Fitness on the Road

Traveling can be a challenge to any workout routine, but there's usually a way to fit in at least some vigorous exercise. The key is to remember that you're working out because of how it makes you feel. Picture how energized and relaxed you are after a workout, how clearheaded and alert, how patient and ready to tackle even the toughest problem. Why wouldn't you want to give yourself those benefits while on a business trip or even a pleasure excursion? In the old days, when you drank coffee, wouldn't you have taken fifteen minutes to walk into a coffee shop, wait in line, and buy your caffeinated boost of energy? You can take the same fifteen minutes to work out, with even better results. The key is to view it as a choice and not just one more obligation.

Sample Situation Visualizations

You're on a business trip in a strange city. Your plane gets in at 8 P.M., and you have an 8 A.M. breakfast the next morning, with back-to-back-meetings for the next two days.

Sample visualization: I see myself asking the woman at the check-in desk about the neighborhood here. I tell her I'd like to take a walk in the morning, and she gets out a map and shows me a route I might take.

Then I go into my hotel room and unpack. It's now about 9 o'clock. I've brought my favorite essential oils with me, and my dry-brush. As soon as I've unpacked, I go into the bathroom and start the water running. While the tub is filling, I brush myself vigorously, then soak in the tub. I can smell the grapefuit and cypress . . . mmmmmm! I feel relaxed and my skin is glowing from the brushing. I sit at the table in my hotel room in my night-gown and take an hour to go over my notes for the next day. Then I get into bed with my favorite airplane reading, read for fifteen minutes, and sleep deeply for eight hours.

The next morning, I put on my workout clothes as soon as I get out of bed. I take the elevator down to the lobby, holding the map that the desk clerk made for me. There's only time for a fifteen-minute walk, but I push myself to move as briskly as I can. I start out feeling sluggish, but by the end of my workout, I feel energized and awake. I go upstairs, shower, put on the clothes I laid out the night before, and head off to my breakfast meeting.

Your sister, her husband, and their kids are coming for the weekend. You know from past visits that it's very difficult to plan anything while they're here, because the three children each seem to have different schedules and interests.

Sample visualization: I see myself talking to my sister on the phone the week before the visit. I'm telling her that I've started this new fitness routine, that it's really important for my health, and that I'd love to work in an hour each day where I can slip off and do my exercise. Does she have any thoughts about when it might work best for me to do this? Does one of her kids have a regular naptime? Maybe I could use the naptime for my workout time.

Here are some tips for combining the Fat Flush Fitness Plan with your life on the road. We can tell you from experience that they work, because with our busy travel schedules, we've had to try them all! We can also tell you that the key to these can be summed up in four words: *be flexible and forgiving.* If you try to duplicate your home workout entirely, of course you're going to fail. If you beat yourself up for doing fifteen minutes of cardio instead of thirty, you won't do any at all and will probably find yourself reaching for a caffeine-and-sugar lift instead. But if you continually congratulate yourself for nurturing your body with the exercise it needs, you'll be surprised at how much you can accomplish, even on the most demanding trip.

Tips for Combining Workout and Travel

- Pack your strength ball, tubing, or bands—or buy some inflatable weights. None of these items are heavy and they take very little space to pack. The inflatable weights are filled with water and can weigh up to 16 pounds.
- If you're taking a road trip, bring your rebounder. A fold-up rebounder will fit in the trunk of your car.
- Try to get up and stretch every hour on a plane, and to take regular hourly breaks during a car trip. Movement keeps your lymphatic system flowing and flushes out toxins. Of course, you can't always move around on a plane the way you'd like, but at least kick off your shoes and wiggle your toes periodically to keep the circulation flowing. If you're concerned about varicose veins, you can buy special support socks that keep the blood flowing toward your heart.
- Drink lots of water when you fly. It's very dehydrating to be in a plane, and the long hours of sitting allow lots of waste products and toxins to build up within your system. Flush them out with a good deal of water. We like to carry several bottles of water on the plane to keep from pestering the flight attendants.
- Ask the desk clerk or concierge what facilities the hotel has to offer. Most hotels these days have fitness rooms, with maybe a treadmill and some weights. You might also schedule a massage during your visit! If the hotel massage therapist can perform a lymphatic drainage massage, terrific. But even a regular massage is good for your circulation and your lymphatic system—and it's a great stress releaser on a difficult trip.
- Rent a fitness video or DVD from the hotel. Many hotels have DVD players or VCRs in every room, and you'd be surprised at how many in-room fitness routines you can do.

- Ask the desk clerk or concierge where you can take a walk. A brisk walk in the morning, or at the end of the afternoon when you feel drained, can help rev you up for the challenging work ahead.
- Get in short walks wherever you can. Instead of trying to block out forty minutes for a full cardio workout, wear or carry comfortable shoes and take advantage of little bits of time. Most hub airports require ten minutes just to change planes. Many office buildings have accessible stairways. A little movement will help you blow off the tension that often accompanies business meetings and enable you to stay clear, calm, and focused.
- Start your day with the Sun Salutation. And throw in a Sun Salutation when you're changing from day to evening clothes. This total body stretching exercise will help relax you like nothing else, bringing healthful oxygen to your brain and getting your blood moving. It only takes five minutes, and it leaves you feeling great. Imagine a business trip on which you did a Sun Salutation in the morning, one while you were changing into your evening wear, and one more about ninety minutes before bedtime. Just those three five-minute intervals can make a huge difference in how you feel.
- If you're visiting friends or family, ask for their help. As you plan your time together, let your loved ones know that you'd like to fit in thirty minutes or an hour to take a brisk walk or to do some strength training. If you let them know ahead of time what you need, they can work your fitness time into plans for the visit.

Take It Easy

As you think about taking your fitness routine on the road, remember that it's not the end of the world if you miss a day or two, or if you cut back on the number of minutes you're "supposed" to work out. What's more important is that you stay active—not because we said so, but because your body will feel better if you do. If you've already started exercising, you've probably noticed that a vigorous workout helps melt away tension as well as fat, bringing oxygen to your brain and getting your blood moving. Even a little movement can bring you these benefits, and staying active even to a lesser extent will definitely make it easier to resume your routine when you get back home. So be kind to yourself, whether that means forgoing some exercise, making an extra effort to keep your routine going, or both.

Fitness and Vacation

Hey, it's vacation. Finally, the time that's supposed to be all about you. The best thing you can do for yourself is exactly what you feel like doing.

But, we hope by now that what you feel like doing includes being active, at least to some extent. This is your chance to try some new things—dancing, snorkeling, walks in new cities or landscapes, horseback riding. Even if you're not on a vacation that lends itself to physical activity, sneaking in some time for a brisk walk and a Sun Salutation will keep you feeling energized and at the top of your form. After all, who wants to feel bloated and sluggish on a vacation? Keeping your muscles active, your lymph and your blood flowing, and your brain well supplied with oxygen will only enhance your pleasure, no matter what kind of vacation you're taking.

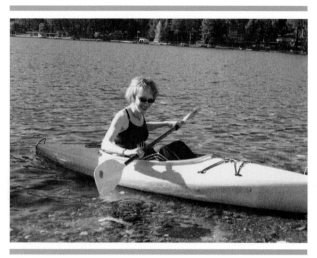

Tips for Staying Active on Vacation

- Start the day with a Sun Salutation. Nothing beats this exercise for total body awareness—a pleasure in your physical self that will make the rest of your day even more fun.
- If you're not doing any other physical activity, build in some brisk walks. Beaches, cities, even hotel casinos offer lots of opportunities for walking quickly and energetically, your arms and legs pumping, your lymph flowing. Just fifteen to twenty minutes can give you energy that will last the rest of your day and evening.
- Take your essential oils and your dry brush. When better to soak in a tub than on vacation? And that dry-brush massage is a great pick-me-up for the transition time between afternoon and evening.
- If you're traveling with a companion, ask him or her to give you the Lymph-Pump massage. So it's not the most romantic thing in the world to do—but it will keep you feeling energized, which can have other romantic benefits. And if you're traveling with a friend, he or she will appreciate the chance to do something that's so good for your health.

We all have trouble staying on track during the holidays. It's not just a question of eating plans and fitness routines—the holidays seem to throw an emotional monkey wrench into everybody's lives. Experts agree that holiday periods can be highly stressful, partly because we all have such intense expectations about what these times are supposed to mean for us.

Likewise, no matter how much fun it may be hosting or being hosted, both being a guest and receiving guests can be stressful as well as pleasurable. The very things that lead us to welcome changes in our routine can also bring added pressure into our lives.

So once again our advice to you is double sided. On one hand, it's fine if you give yourself a bit of a break during the holidays. You probably won't stick to your eating and fitness plans as well as you might during the rest of the year—and why should you? Life would get pretty boring if you did the same exact thing 365 days a year. By the same token, there's nothing wrong with modifying your diet and lifestyle while hosting guests or on a visit.

On the other hand, if you see healthy eating and regular exercise as part of how you take care of yourself, why should you give it up just because it's a holiday, or because loved ones have come to see you? It may be challenging to find new ways of handling visits, holidays, and other social occasions, but if the stakes are your sense of well-being and physical comfort, it's worth putting in the effort.

Tips for Handling Holidays, Visits, and Special Occasions

- Visualize the entire event. Picture yourself arriving at a friend's home, for example, and eating the food she serves. Given your new eating habits, how will you feel when the meal is over? Satisfied? Bloated? Frustrated that you've eaten "toxic" foods? Happy because it all tastes so good? Likewise, imagine the day you have a big holiday party to attend, a party that tempts you into skipping your workout routine. How will you feel when the day is over? Glowing with the pleasure of the party? Tense and frustrated because your muscles haven't been used? Imagining the entire event will help you choose what you need to do to make everything work for you.
- Be as matter-of-fact as possible about what you need. If you were allergic to, say, peanuts, you simply wouldn't eat them, right? You wouldn't politely eat a big handful, and then ask your hostess to take

you to the emergency room. You can treat your new eating and fitness needs exactly the same way. Figure out what you must tell other people about, and what you can simply handle on your own. The more casual and yet committed you are, the easier it will be to continue with the activities and eating habits you've chosen.

- Remember that the *Fat Flush Cookbook* offers lots of fabulous recipes. The whole point is for no one to feel deprived. If you're hosting friends and family, you could probably go a whole weekend without anyone even noticing that you're eating differently—though you might get lots of compliments on your cooking!

Fitness for the New You

Emily, whom we met in Chapter 1, was delighted with the changes she had made in her life. Going on the Fat Flush eating and fitness plans had enabled her to lose weight, gain boundless energy, and feel better than she had in years. This busy ER nurse found she had more patience with her children, more energy for her patients, and more joy and optimism about herself.

"I think it's great," she told us. "But I've got to admit, sometimes I get worried about how long it will last. I've been pretty good about staying on track so far. But what happens in a year, or two years? I'm not so sure I'll be able to keep this routine up, just because that's the way life seems to go."

"Well," Joanie told her, "I've met hundreds of women who have attended my fit camps. Lots of them check back with me after a few months or even a few years. And here's what I've noticed: the ones who stick with staying fit are the ones who keep making changes in their lives. Now that fitness has made so many new things possible for them, they keep going forward, trying new things, developing new goals. My sense is that in life, there's no such thing as staying in the same place. You're either moving forward or you're slipping backward."

Emily thought about this for a moment and nodded. "Okay," she said. "I guess I've achieved all the goals I set for myself when I started this plan. Now maybe it's time to set some new goals."

As we approach the end of this book, that's the best advice we could possibly give you: when you've achieved your fitness goals, set some more. Your new goals won't necessarily involve fitness per se. Maybe, now that you're feeling so healthy and energized, you'd like to learn a new language, or go back to school for an advanced degree. Maybe you'd like to become a Big

Sister or a foster parent. Perhaps you've always wanted to learn to weave. Or maybe the other day you were passing by an airfield and it suddenly hit you—you'd like to learn how to fly a plane.

None of these goals are directly related to weight, health, and fitness. But that's the point—your health, fitness, and new levels of energy are for you to use in any way you choose. We hope that staying fit and active will always be a part of your life—because it broadens all your choices while keeping you in touch with the simple pleasure of being alive.

So take a moment to envision some new aspect of your existence. Then write a pledge in which you tell yourself how you plan to bring it into your life. If you keep coming back to this process again and again, you'll be enjoying the best recipe for happiness we could ever share with you.

My New Desire:

_____

_____

_____

_____

_____

_____

_____

_____

_____

_____

_____

_____

_____

My New Pledge:

_____

_____

_____

_____

_____

_____

_____

_____

_____

_____

_____

_____

_____

_____

_____

_____

_____

_____

_____

_____

_____

_____

_____

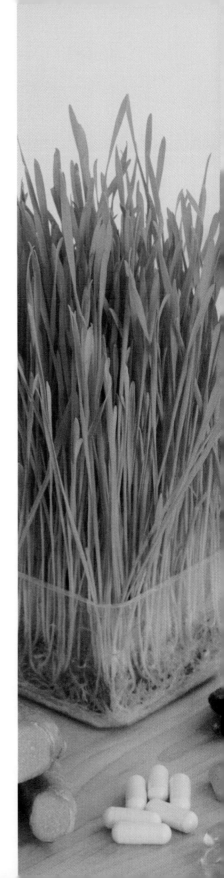

10
General Fat Flush Support and Resources

Go where life takes you. You may be surprised at what it gives.

—AUTHOR UNKNOWN

Here are some of the most reliable and solid resources for a variety of fitness-related areas ranging from Fat Flush support, to some of the best equipment sources, to specialty items, clothing suppliers, videos, Web sites, books, and organizations with superior products and useful information for achieving overall health and fitness.

Fat Flush Support and Resources

On the Web: www.fatflush.com and www.joaniegreggains.com

We invite you to check out both of our Web sites. On fatflush.com, you will now find a Fat Flush store that is updated regularly with all the dietary products that have the Fat Flush seal of approval: the Fat Flush Kit (the Dieter's Multi, GLA 90, and the Weight Loss Formula); Fat Flush Whey Protein Powder, Flaxseed Oil, Health from the Sun High-Lignan Flaxseed Oil capsules, flaxseed grinders, the Woman's Oil, CLA 1000, Ultra H-3 (for depression), Y-C Cleanse (for yeast control), Super GI Cleanse, Dandelion

Root Tea, and Teeccino (the herbal coffee substitute). Ann Louise's calendar is updated regularly on this site so you can keep track of her media events, lectures, and radio and TV appearances.

On Joanie's site, you will find health and fitness articles, a health tip of the week, and information on how to order her DVDs and CDs. This site will be updated continually with Joanie's latest appearances and promotional schedules.

On the Web: www.fatflush.com/forum

And of course, you are most cordially invited to become part of our Fat Flush Forum, where special fitness questions can be posted. This forum is supported by outstanding veteran Fat Flush community leaders who are constantly in touch with both Ann Louise and Joanie. On this forum, you can have your Fat Flush Fitness questions answered and be the first to know of the latest fitness updates.

As another convenience for Ann Louise's many readers and clients, Uni Key Health Systems has been the official distributor of Fat Flush and related health care products, books, and services over the years. Uni Key is the fulfillment center for Ann Louise's online store and the only official distributor of the Fat Flush Kit and Fat Flush brand products. Contact Uni Key directly if you would prefer to speak with a "live" customer service representative. Their telephone number is 800-888-4353

General Tips for Buying Exercise Equipment

- Determine your goals. Look for a program that fits your needs.
- Will you really use exercise equipment? Before you buy, prove to yourself that you're ready to stick to an ongoing fitness program.
- No piece of equipment can help you spot reduce. There is no such thing as "spot reducing," since you can not burn fat off a particular part of your body.
- Be aware of outrageous claims. Claims that promise "easy" or effortless" results are false.
- Check the fine print. Look for tipoffs that getting the "advertised results" requires more than just using the machine.
- Try equipment before you buy. Get details on warranties, guarantees, return policies, and customer service.

EXERCISE EQUIPMENT

REBOUNDERS/MINITRAMPOLINES

Jumpking Trampolines

Clark and Associates
10016a Royal Lane
Dallas, TX 75238
800-488-0466
214-342-0919
www.jumpright.com

This company boasts that it is the world's largest manufacturer of trampolines, and rebounders.

MegaFitness

P.O. Box 33536
Melbourne, FL 32903
800-925-2772 (order line)
321-674-3866 (customer service)
www.megafitness.com

This online store sells high-quality fitness equipment (personal trampolines) and accessories.

Needak Manufacturing

P.O. Box 776
O'Neill, NE 68763
800-232-5762
402-336-4083
www.needakrebounders.com

Founded in 1990, this company is the only firm that manufactures its own rebounders in the United States. The Needak Soft-Bounce is the best-selling model for at-home use. The company also offers folding travel rebounders for easy packing in a car trunk. The stabilizing bar is optional for those individuals who desire more balancing support. (Do let the company know that Fat Flush sent you.)

ReboundAIR

American Institute of Reboundology, Inc.
520 South Commerce Drive
Orem, UT 84058
888-464-JUMP (5867)
www.reboundair.com

Founded by Al Carter, the original pioneer of rebounding in this country, this company is one of the leaders in rebounder minitrampolines. With no assembly required, the ReboundAIR is portable and can be folded in half for transport. There is also a quarter-fold model available, convenient for airline travelers, with a custom-fitted carrying case and a free pull dolly. The lifetime warranty comes with a free wear-and-tear replacement. The stabilizing bar is sold separately and can be fitted to any model. (If you order from this company, tell them Fat Flush sent you.)

Stamina Pro Jogger

Stamina Customer Service
P.O. Box 1071
Springfield, MO 65801-1071
800-375-7520
www.staminafitness.com

Stamina products are also available in selected retail stores, in 48-inch, all-steel frame construction, with a stabilizing bar and a 250-pound weight limit.

Super Tramp

Langlands Business Park
Uffculme
Culompton
Devon
EX15 3DA
www.supertramp.co.uk
sales@supertramp.co.uk

A UK company, Super Tramp provides rebounders that are designed and built to be left outside year round.

STRENGTH BALLS

JumpUSA

1290 Lawrence Station Road
Sunnyvale, CA 94089
800-586-7872
www.jumpusa.com

This company sells the special plyoballs used in the Fat Flush Strength Ball Workout, available in different sizes, from 1 to 30 pounds.

DUMBBELLS

AquaBells Dumbbells and Ankle Weights

6060 Gallagher Road
Pilot Hill, CA 95664
800-987-6892
www.aquabells.com

Totally portable and collapsible, these dumbbells and ankle weights are the perfect solution for weight training on the road, or even at home.

Fogdog Sports

P.O. Box 489
Melbourne, FL 32902-0489
800-624-2017
www.fogdog.com

This online store is a great source of fitness equipment, sporting goods, and apparel.

CONSUMER RESOURCES

www.exercise-equipment-review.com

This Web site offers informative, straight-to-the-point articles on fitness equipment, featuring products seen on television.

ConsumerSearch

> 5467 31st Street NW
> Washington, DC 20015
> 202-966-7907
> www.consumersearch.com

This Internet-based publishing company helps consumers find answers about top-rated products based on research articles about any given product or service; the references are then analyzed and ranked for credibility.

DVD/VIDEO, CDS, CLOTHING, AND FITNESS ACCESSORIES

Bodytrends.com

> 6385-B Rose Lane
> Carpinteria, CA 93013
> 800-549-1667
> www.bodytrends.com/pbelt.htm

This company carries a wide variety of fitness equipment and offers comparison charts.

Collage Video

> 5390 Main Street NE
> Minneapolis, MN 55421-1128
> 800-433-6769
> www.collagevideo.com

This company has a great selection of workout videos, geared to the beginner as well as to the ultra-advanced.

Fitness Wholesale

> Future Dynamics Division
> 895-A Hampshire Road
> Stow, OH 44224
> 888-FW-ORDER
> 330-929-7227
> www.fitnesswholesale.com

In addition to Thera-Band and Challenge PRO products, Fitness Wholesale supplies a full line of fitness equipment accessories, including resistance bands and tubing, weights, mats, charts, videos, aquatic products, fitness balls, balance aids, and more, all at wholesale prices.

Foot Smart

P.O. Box 922908
Norcross, GA 30010-2908
800-870-7149
www.footsmart.com

This is an online store/catalog company offering comfort footwear and health care products for the lower body.

Joanie Greggains

P.O. Box 2708
Sausalito, CA 94966
415-332-8566
www.joaniegreggains.com

Great selections of Joanie's workout DVD/videos to complement the Fat Flush Fitness Plan. Also offers videos that target specific areas, such as a walking CD—perfect for all Fat Flushers.

Polar Heart Monitor

Polar Electro, Inc.
370 Crossways Park Drive
Woodbury, NY 11797-2050
800-227-1314
www.polarusa.com

Polar heart rate monitors are designed to provide you with up-to-the-minute heart rate feedback—ideal for anyone striving to achieve her optimum Fat Flush fitness personal best.

Thor-Lo, Inc.

2210 Newton Drive
Statesville, NC 28677
800-438-0209
704-872-6522
www.thorlo.com (to locate a dealer)

Thor-Lo socks are the perfect accessory to meet the demands of walking or any other sport or activity. The varying densities of padding help to protect from foot pain.

WristWand

> PMB 246
> 336 Bon Air Center
> Greenbrae, CA 94904
> 800-681-9762
> 415-457-7990
> www.wristwand.com

The Wrist Wand is a unique portable device that stretches areas commonly under stress, such as the medial tendons and ligaments of the wrist from routine use of the computer keyboard. Tennis players and musicians can also benefit from its use.

LIFESTYLE RESOURCES

Meridian Sports Club Rolling Hills Novato

> 351 San Andreas Drive
> Novato, CA 94945
> 415-897-2185
> www.meridiansportsclubs.com

A full-service sports club whose mission is to provide an environment of health and fitness through sports recreation, wellness, and rehabilitation.

SKIN CARE

> American Academy of Dermatology
> P.O. Box 4014
> 847-330-0230
> www.aad.org

American Academy of Dermatology serves as a source of information on dermatology, providing resourcs on healthy skin issues and a free e-newsletter.

Jakaré Natural Skin Care

> P.O. Box 10124
> Bozeman, MT 59719-0124
> 1-877-JAKARE1 (1-877-525-2731)
> www.jakare.com

This company specializes in aromatherapy-based skin care using pure organic essential oils made fresh weekly. They provide a range of products to accommodate all skin types, with an emphasis on antiaging and restoring youthful skin vitality naturally. Jakare also offers exceptional carrier oils for custom blending and moisturizing for the body.

AROMATHERAPY

North American Herb & Spice Company

Internatural
P.O. Box 4885
Buffalo Grove, IL 60089
800-243-5242
www.internatural-alternative-health.com

This company is renowned for its exceptionally pure and therapeutic wild oregano oil, which can be used both internally and topically for myriad health challenges including Candida, parasites, bacteria, virues, and chemical poisoning. In addition, it has many other essential oils that also can be used therapeutically.

Tisserand Aromatherapy

Newton Road
Hove
Sussex, BN3 7BA
44 1273 325666
44 1273 208444 (fax)
e-mail: info@avalonnaturalproducts.com (USA & Canada)
www.tisserand.com

Tisserand Aromatherapy offers over fifty pure essential oils, including a limited organic collection, that are suitable for bathing, vaporization, and massage.

Young Living Essentials

250 South Main Street
Payson, UT 84651
800-371-3515
801-465-5424 (fax)
www.youngliving.com

Founded in 1993, Young Living Essential Oils is renowned for exceptionally high-quality essential oils.

FITNESS AND HEALTH ORGANIZATIONS

Allhealth.com

Allhealth.com is the health site of ivillage.com, the women's network.

American College of Sports Medicine (ACSM)

> P.O. Box 1440
> Indianapolis, IN 46206-1440
> 317-637-9200 (national center)
> www.acsm.org

A large part of ACSM's mission is devoted to public awareness and education about the positive aspects of physical activity for people of all ages, from all walks of life. A great resource for information with articles, brochures, and recommendations available through the Web site.

American Council on Exercise (ACE)

> 4851 Paramount Drive
> San Diego, California 92123
> 800-825-3636
> 858-279-8227
> www.acefitness.com

ACE not only sets the standards for fitness professionals and provides rigorous testing to assure those standards are met, but also serves as the leading nonprofit fitness advocate. The ACE Web site is a great resource for safe and effective exercise.

American Diabetes Association

> ATTN: National Call Center
> 1701 North Beauregard Street
> Alexandria, VA 22311
> 800-342-2383
> www.diabetes.org

The American Diabetes Association is the nation's leading nonprofit health organization providing diabetes research, information, and advocacy. The mission of the organization is to prevent and cure diabetes and to improve the lives of all people affected by it. Resources, information, and a free newsletter are available.

AFAA (Aerobics and Fitness Association of America)

15250 Ventura Boulevard, Suite 200
Sherman Oaks, CA 91403-3297
800-968-7263 (consumer hotline)
800-446-2322
www.afaa.com

The Aerobics and Fitness Association of America is the world's largest fitness and TeleFitness Educator. Founded in 1983, AFAA has certified more than 150,000 instructors from seventy-three countries. Led by a distinguished group of health and fitness advisors, AFAA produces a wide variety of educational materials, including *American Fitness* magazine, textbooks, reference manuals, and videos. Each year, AFAA puts on over 2,500 educational workshops.

Arthritis Foundation

P.O. Box 7669
Atlanta, GA 30357-0669
800-283-7800
www.arthritis.org

The Arthritis Foundation is the only national, not-for-profit organization that supports the more than one hundred types of arthritis and related conditions with advocacy, programs, services, and research.

The Cooper Institute

12330 Preston Road
Dallas, TX 75230
972-341-3200
courses@cooperinst.org

The Cooper Institute is dedicated to advancing the understanding of the relationship between living habits and health and to providing leadership in implementing these concepts to enhance the physical and emotional well-being of individuals.

Food and Drug Administration (FDA)

5600 Fisher's Lane
Rockville, MD 20857
888-info-fda
http://www.fda.gov

The FDA oversees pharmaceuticals as well as medical devices, and their approval.

healthfinder®

> P.O. Box 1133
> Washington, DC 20013-1133
> Healthfinder
> www.healthfinder.gov

Healthfinder was developed by the U.S. Department of Health and Human Services together with other federal agencies to provide a key resource for finding the best government and nonprofit health and human services information on the Internet, including online publications, clearinghouses, databases, Web sites, and support and self-help groups.

InteliHealth

> www.intellihealth.com

Provides information drawn from reliable sources, featuring Harvard Medical School's consumer health information.

LifeMatters

> 1275 4th Street
> Santa Rosa, CA 95401
> 888-255-9757
> www.lifematters.com

Products and online classes providing resources to help people take charge of their health and well-being.

Medem

> 649 Mission Street, 2nd Floor
> San Francisco, CA 94105
> 877-926-3336
> www.medem.com

Medem's award-winning consumer information comes from the combined libraries of forty-four of the nation's leading medical societies, the organizations that doctors trust most. The library holds more than four thousand peer-reviewed articles and helps patients navigate subjects from introductory to advanced-level materials. To ensure medical accuracy, existing articles are updated regularly and new ones are added every week.

National Osteoporosis Foundation

1232 22nd Street NW
Washington, DC 20037-1292
800-223-9994
202-223 2226
www.nof.org

The National Osteoporosis Foundation (NOF) is the leading nonprofit, voluntary health organization dedicated to promoting lifelong bone health in order to reduce the widespread prevalence of osteoporosis and associated fractures, while working to find a cure for the disease through research, education, and advocacy.

Sara's City Workout

1617 Orrington Avenue, Suite 202
Evanston, IL 60201
800-545-CITY
www.saracity.com

Sara's City Workout is the leader in fitness-instructor education and the largest provider of continuing education credits (CECs) for group exercise instructors, aquatic professionals, and personal trainers offering cutting-edge conventions, certifications,

RxList—The Internet Drug Index

500 3rd Street, Suite 530
San Francisco, CA 94107
www.rxlist.com

A very useful drug index with information for both consumers and professionals.

WebMD

1-877-GO-WEBMD
www.webmd.com

WebMD Health is a consumer-focused health care information Web site providing information that helps people play an active role in managing their own health.

NUTRITION EDUCATION

American College of Nutrition
300 South Duncan Avenue, Suite 225
Clearwater, FL 33755
727- 446-6086
e-mail: office@am-coll-nutr.org

The American College of Nutrition was established in 1959 to promote scientific endeavor in the field of nutritional sciences.

FAT FLUSH BOOKS

Here is a listing and a brief description of books that are excellent companions for your Fat Flush journey.

The Fat Flush Plan

Ann Louise Gittleman, M.S., C.N.S.
New York: McGraw-Hill, 2002

The Fat Flush Plan is the *USA Today* and *NY Times* bestseller that melts fat from hips, waist, and thighs in just two weeks and reshapes your body while detoxifying your system.

The Fat Flush Cookbook

Ann Louise Gittleman, M.S., C.N.S.
New York: McGraw-Hill, 2002

The *Fat Flush Cookbook* is the companion cookbook to the national bestseller which offers more than two hundred recipes for fast breakfasts, one dish luncheons and dinners, plus snacks and scrumptious desserts using a wide variety of fat-flushing foods, drinks, and culinary herbs and spices to cleanse and slim the body.

The Fat Flush Journal and Shopping Guide

Ann Louise Gittleman, M.S., C.N.S.
New York: McGraw-Hill, 2003

The Fat Flush Journal and Shopping Guide is your handy, take-anywhere companion to The Fat Flush Plan that helps you to record your progress, weight loss, and future goals. It helps you track meals, supplements, and exercise and inspires you with daily motivational messages.

OTHER BOOKS FOR YOUR BOOKSHELF

Anybody's Sports Medicine Book:
The Complete Guide to Quick Recovery from Injuries
> Dr. James Garrick, Peter Radetsky
> Berkeley, CA: Ten Speed Press, 2000

This book tells you what to do immediately, when to see a doctor and how to rehabilitate your injury. Organized by injured body part, along with rehab exercise illustrations, commonly asked questions as well as tips and special considerations.

Dr. James Garrick heads San Francisco's Center for Sports Medicine and is the medical advisor to the National Football League, the U.S. Olympic Figure Skating Team and the San Francisco Ballet.

Exercising Through Your Pregnancy
> James F. Clapp III, M.D.
> Champaign, IL: Human Kinetics, 1998

Dr. Clapp, the leading authority on exercise and pregnancy, summarizes all the latest research and provides hands-on guidance for before, during, and after pregnancy in a very reassuring style.

Fit Happens
> Joanie Greggains (with Patricia Romanowski)
> New York: Villard Books, 1999

Fitness isn't a job or an obligation. It's the natural result of making good positive lifestyle choices every day. *Fit Happens* shows you how.

The Fitness Factor
> Lisa Callahan, M.D.
> Guilford, CT: The Lyons Press, 2002

Based on Dr. Callahan's work as the founder of the Women's Sports Medicine Center at the Hospital for Special Surgery in New York, this book offers practical advice for incorporating fitness into your life, with simple drawings illustrating her routines.

Jonny Bowden's Shape Up

> Jonny Bowden, M.A., C.N., C.N.S.
> Cambridge, MA: Perseus, 2001

Jonny Bowden, iVillage's successful "Weight Loss Coach," helps you design an eating program for yourself that is personalized for your measurements, temperament, lifestyle, and metabolic and biochemical uniqueness.

Jonny Bowden's Shape Up Workbook

> Jonny Bowden, M.A., C.N., C.N.S.
> Cambridge, MA: Perseus, 2002

A diet and workout log packed with recipes, training tips, and inspiration.

The Living Beauty Detox Program

> Ann Louise Gittleman, M.S., C.N.S.
> San Francisco: Harper, 2000

The Living Beauty Detox Program helps women of all ages determine their seasonal type using specially designed quizzes, and offers regimens to resolve the problems that can plague women of every beauty type. Here you will find the beauty fundamentals every woman needs to maintain a healthier, more radiant appearance.

Strong Women Stay Young (revised edition)

> Miriam E. Nelson, Ph.D., with Sarah Wernick, Ph.D.
> New York: Bantam Books, 2002

This illustrated book, based on Dr. Nelson's extensive research on the effects of exercise on women and the elderly, offers real-world advice on making exercise a part of your life.

Yoga for Beginners

> Mark Ansari and Liz Lark
> New York: HarperCollins, 1998

Full-color photographs throughout, a handy hands-free format, and programs designed for both beginning and intermediate-level exercisers make this a useful guide for those relatively new to yoga.

Notes

Preface

1. Gary Taubes, "What If It's All Been a Big Fat Lie?," *New York Times*, July 7, 2002, sec.6.

2. Katherine M. Flegal, et al., "Prevalence and Trends in Obesity Among U.S. Adults, 1999–2000," *Journal of the American Medical Association* 288 (October 9, 2002): 1726.

Introduction

1. Ann Louise Gittleman, *The Fat Flush Plan* (New York: McGraw-Hill, 2002), 20.

2. S. E. Taylor, et al., "Biobehavioral Responses to Stress in Females: Tend-and-Befriend, not Fight-or-Flight," *Psychological Review* 107 (July 2000), 745–50.

Chapter 1

1. Ann Louise Gittleman, *The Fat Flush Plan* (New York: McGraw-Hill, 2002), 11–39.

2. R. J. Williams III, et al., "The Effect of Ciprofloxacin on Tendon, Paratenon, and Capsular Fibroblast Metabolism," *American Journal of Sports Medicine* 28 (May 2000): 364–69.

3. Gittleman, *Fat Flush*, 20.

4. Ibid., 29–30.

5. Elizabeth Dancey, *The Cellulite Solution* (New York: St. Martin's Press, 1996), 19.

6. Hans Selye, *The Stress of Life*, rev. ed. (New York: McGraw-Hill, 1984).

7. P. Peeke and G. P. Chrousos, "Hypercortisolism and Obesity," *Annals of the New York Academy of Science* 771 (December 29, 1995): 665–76.

8. Gittleman, *Fat Flush*, 36–7.

9. Ibid., 37–8.

10. JoAnn E. Manson, et al., "Physical Activity and Incidence of Coronary Heart Disease and Stroke in Females," *Circulation* 91 (1995): 927.

11. JoAnn E. Manson, et al., "Walking Compared with Vigorous Exercise for the Prevention of Cardiovascular Events in Women," *New England Journal of Medicine* 347 (September 5, 2002): 722–3.

12. Nanci Helmich, "Health Is Just Steps Away: Even Moderate Activity Can Bring Significant Benefits, Expert Says," *USA Today*, November 23, 2002, D9.

13. D. Feskanich, W. Willett, and G. Colditz, "Walking and Leisure-Time Activity and Risk of Hip Fracture in Postmenopausal Women," *Journal of the American Medical Association* 288 (November 13, 2002): 2300.

14. Nanci Helmich, "Health Is Just Steps Away: Exercise Cuts Risk of Hip Fractures," *USA Today*, November 13, 2002, D9.

15. Gerald M. Lemole, *The Healing Diet* (New York: William Morrow, 2001), 160.

Chapter 2

1. Gittleman, *Fat Flush*, 103–4.

2. S. J. Colcombe, et al., "Aerobic Fitness Reduces Brain Tissue Loss in Aging Humans," *Journal of Gerontology Series A: Biological Science and Medical Science* 58 (February 2003): 176–80.

Chapter 3

1. Eugenia E. Calle, et al., "Overweight, Obesity, and Mortality from Cancer in a Prospectively Studied Cohort of U.S. Adults," *New England Journal of Medicine* 348 (April 24, 2003): 1625.

2. Ibid.

3. Katherine M. Flegal, et al., "Prevalence and Trends in Obesity Among U.S. Adults, 1999-2000," *Journal of the American Medical Association* 288 (October 9, 2002): 1726.

4. Helene Glassberg and Gary J. Balady, "Exercise and Heart Disease in Women: Why, How, and How Much?" *Cardiology in Review* 7 (September 1999): 301.

5. Marcia L. Stefanick, et al., "Effects of Diet and Exercise in Men and Postmenopausal Women with Low Levels of HDL Cholesterol and High Levels of LDL Cholesterol," *New England Journal of Medicine* 339 (July 1998): 12.

6. J. L. Durstine, et al., "Lipids, Lipoproteins, and Exercise," *Journal of Cardiopulmonary Rehabilitation* 22 (November 2002): 385.

7. Well-Connected Web site, "What Are the Effects of Exercise on the Heart and Circulation?" www.well-connected.com/report.cgi/000029_3.htm (accessed July 3, 2003).

8. Jeffrey L. Tanji, "The Benefits of Exercise for Women," *Clinics in Sports Medicine* 19 (April 2000): 175–85.

9. A. M. de Diego Acosta, et al., "Influence of Fitness on the Integrated Neuroendocrine Response to Aerobic Exercise Until Exhaustion," *Journal of Physiology and Biochemistry* 57 (December 2001): 313–20.

10. Albert E. Carter, *The New Miracles of Rebound Exercise*, rev. ed. (Edmonds, WA: The National Institute of Reboundology and Health, 1988), 166.

11. A. Bhattacharya, et al., "Body Acceleration Distribution and O2 Uptake in Humans During Running and Jumping," *Journal of Applied Physiology* 49 (November 1980): 881–7.

12. Gerald M. Lemole, *The Healing Diet* (New York: William Morrow, 2001), 160.

13. Ibid.

14. Colleen A. McGlone, Len Kravitz, and Jeffrey M. Janot, "Rebounding: A Low-Impact Exercise Alternative," www.urbanrebounding.com/benefits.html (accessed June 9, 2003).

15. Y. Mutoh, et al., "Aerobic Dance Injuries Among Instructors and Students," *Physician and Sportsmedicine* 16 (February 1988): 81–83.

16. U.S. Department of Health and Human Services, *Physical Activity and Health: A Report of the Surgeon General* (Atlanta, GA: Centers for Disease Control and Prevention, National Center for Chronic Disease Prevention and Health Promotion, 1996).

17. J. R. Stofan, et al., "Physical Activity Patterns Associated with Cardiorespiratory Fitness and Reduced Mortality: The Aerobics Center Longitudinal Study," *American Journal of Public Health* 88 (December 1998): 1807–13.

18. U.S. Dept. of Health, *Physical Activity*.

19. JoAnn E. Manson, et al., "Walking Compared with Vigorous Exercise for the Prevention of Cardiovascular Events in Women," *New England Journal of Medicine* 347 (September 5, 2002): 721.

Chapter 4

1. Maria A. Fiatarone Singh, "Exercise to Prevent and Treat Functional Disability," *Clinics in Geriatric Medicine* 18 (2002): 437.

2. Wayne Westcott and Rita La Rosa Loud, *No More Cellulite* (New York: Perigee, 2003), 13–5.

3. Michael R. Deschenes and William J. Kraemer, "Performance and Physiologic Adaptations to Resistance Training," *American Journal of Physical Medicine & Rehabilitation* 81 (2002): S3–16.

Chapter 5

1. Elizabeth Dancey, *The Cellulite Solution* (New York: St. Martin's Press, 1996), 48–9.

2. Ibid., 50–1.

Chapter 7

1. M. A. Diego, et al., "HIV Adolescents Show Improved Immune Function Following Massage Therapy," *International Journal of Neuroscience* 106 (January 2001): 35–45.

2. Alan R. Hirsch and R. Gomez, "Weight Reduction Through Inhalation of Odorants," *Journal of Neurology, Orthopedic Medicine and Surgery* 16 (1995): 26–31.

3. Jane Buckle, "The Use of Aromatherapy as a Complementary Treatment of Chronic Pain," *Alternative Therapies in Health and Medicine* 5 (September 1999): 42–51.

4. Jane Buckle, *Clinical Aromatherapy in Nursing* (San Diego, CA: Singular Publishing Group, 1997), 46.

5. *Essential Oils Desk Reference*, 2nd ed. (Salem, UT: Essential Science Publishing, 2001).

6. Joseph Dispenza, *Live Better Longer: The Parcells Center 7-Step Plan for Health and Longevity* (San Francisco: Harper, 1997), 31.

7. L. Redwine, et al., "Effects of Sleep and Sleep Deprivation on Inter-leukin-6, Growth Hormone, Cortisol, and Melatonin Levels in Humans," *Journal of Clinical Endocrinology and Metabolism* 85 (October 2000): 3597–3603.

8. K. Spiegel, R. Leproult, and E. Van Cauter, "Impact of Sleep Debt on Metabolic and Endocrine Function," *The Lancet* 354 (October 23, 1999): 1435–9.

9. E. Van Cauter, R. Leproult, and L. Plat, "Age-Related Changes in Slow Wave Sleep and REM Sleep and Relationship with Growth Hormone and Cortisol Levels in Healthy Men," *Journal of the American Medical Association* 284 (August 16, 2000): 861–8.

10. Sleep Foundation, "Backgrounder: Why Sleep Matters," www.sleepfoundation.org/nsaw/pk_background.html (accessed January 21, 2003).

11. Mary Lee Patton and Bob Condor, *Mary Lee's Natural Health & Beauty* (New York: Jeremy P. Tarcher, 2001), 162.

Chapter 8

1. Elizabeth Dancey, *The Cellulite Solution* (New York: St. Martin's Press, 1996), 18–19.

2. Ibid., 17.

3. Ibid., 17.

4. J. Sun, et al., "Antioxidant and Antiproliferative Activities of Common Fruits," *Journal of Agricultural and Food Chemistry* 50 (December 4, 2002):7449–54.

5. T. Lotti, et al., "Proteoglycans in So-Called Cellulite," *International Journal of Dermatology* 29 (May 1990): 272–4.

6. Ann Louise Gittleman, *The Fat Flush Plan* (New York: McGraw-Hill, 2002), 27.

7. M. W. Pariza, Y. Park, and M. E. Cook, "Conjugated Linoleic Acid and the Control of Cancer and Obesity," *Toxicology and Science* 52 (Supplement 1999): 107–10.

8. Wayne Westcott and Rita LaRosa Loud, *No More Cellulite* (New York: Perigee, 2003), 158.

9. C. Pierard-Franchimont, et al., "A Randomized, Placebo-Controlled Trial of Topical Retinol in the Treatment of Cellulite," *American Journal of Clinical Dermatology* 1 (November 2000): 369–74.

Index

dry-brush massage, 24, 25, 97, 163–65

full-body lymphatic massage, 157–63

Lymph Pump massage, 162–63

when to avoid, 158

Massage therapists, finding, 159

McGee-Cooper, Ann, 37

McGlone, Colleen A., 61

Medications, 5

Medicine balls (*See also* Strength balls)

Methionine, 181

Milk thistle, 181

Minitrampolines (*See* Rebounders)

The Miracles of Rebound Exercise (Albert E. Carter), 58

Motivation:
  and defining goals, 152–53
  for keeping on track, 152–53
  self-encouragement, 6
  when getting started, 27–33

Muscle(s):
  contraction of, 80–81
  core, 83, 139
  lack of exercise and loss of, 174
  lean muscle mass, 23, 31, 78, 80–81, 179
  lengthening, 112
  preserving tone of, 32–33
  toning vs. building, 79–80
  (*See also* Strength training)

NASA (National Aeronautics and Space Administration), 60

National Weight Control Registry, 37

Neurotransmitters, 59

Nike, 179

Noradrenaline, 14, 166

Norepinephrine, 14

Nutrient absorption, 10

Nutrition, 10–11

Obesity, 59

Oregon grape root, 181

Osteoporosis, 59, 80

Pacing yourself, 30–31

Parcells, Hazel, 167–69

Pariza, Michael, 178–79

Perceived exertion, 67

Phase 1, 47–74
  aerobic exercise, 57–58
  cool-down stretches, 70–73
  focus of, 47–48
  rebounding, 58, 60–64
  rest and renewal days, 74
  special features of, 21–23
  Sun Salutation, 49–57
  walking, 64–70
  workout calendar, 75–76

Phase 2, 77–107
  cardio workout, 84–85
  cool-down stretching, 86
  coordinating cardio and strength ball, 84, 86
  rest and renewal days, 97
  special features of, 23–24
  strength ball, 83–84
  strength ball cool-down stretches, 93–95
  strength ball exercises, 87–93
  strength ball six-week schedule, 87
  strength training, 79–83
  tips for accomplishing, 96
  workout calendar, 98–100

Phase 3, 101–119
  abdominal exercises, 132–33, 139
  beginning program at, 31
  benefits of, 105
  cardio workout, 105–8
  cool-down stretches after cardio workout, 108
  coordinating cardio and lymph-fit workouts, 108–9
  defining your goals, 148–52
  dumbbell strength training, 126–33
  fitness routine variations, 124–47
  keeping on track, 152–53
  Lymph-Fit cool-down stretches, 117–18
  Lymph-Fit/Compound Strength and Stretching Workout, 109–17
  resistance band strength training, 134–138
  rest and renewal days, 119

special features of, 24–25

stability ball workout, 139–47

staying motivated, 152–53

workout calendar, 120–21

Phenols, 178

Phosphatidylcholine, 181

Plantar fascia, 111

Pledge, 39–41, 192–93

Posture, 104–105, 111

Preservation of skin and muscle tone, 32–33

Proanthocyanidins, 178

Progesterone, 15

Pump massage, 162–163

Questionnaire, Fitness Plan, 34–36

Rebounders:
  choosing, 61–62
  resources for, 197–198

Rebounding, 22, 58, 60–64
  benefits of, 60–62
  choosing between walking and, 58
  do's and don'ts of, 63
  in Phase 1, 62–64
  in Phase 2, 85
  in Phase 3, 106–108
  as preferred choice, 58

Resistance (as stress response), 16

Resistance bands:
  resource for, 200
  workout with, 134–138

Resources, 195–210
  books, 209–210
  consumer, 199–200
  for DVD/video, CDs, clothing/ accessories, 200–202
  for exercise equipment, 197–99
  Fat Flush books, 208
  fitness and health organizations, 204–7
  lifestyle, 202–3

Rest and renewal days:
  Phase 1, 74
  Phase 2, 97
  Phase 3, 119

Retinols, sensitivity to, 180

Schedule:
  for journaling, 37–38
  planning, 29
  strength ball, 87
  (*See also* Workout calendar)
Self-care:
  associating exercise with, 49
  resistance to, 156
Selye, Hans, 13, 16
Skin care:
  preserving tone, 32–33
  resources for, 202–3
Sleep, 48, 168–171
  and baths, 165
  causes of problems with, 171
  suggestions for encouraging,
    169–71
  and weight loss, 12
Slow-twitch muscle fibers, 82
Smoking, 17
Stability ball, 139–47
Static stretch, 70
Strength balls, 23–24, 79, 83–84
  choosing, 83
  cool-down stretches, 93–95
  coordinating cardio workouts
    with, 86
  exercises, 87–93
  resources for, 199
Strength training, 23
  with dumbbells, 126–33
  individual factors in, 82–83
  Lymph-Fit/Compound Strength
    and Stretching Workout,
    109–17

Phase 2, 23–24, 87–93,
Phase 3, 104, 126–38
  with resistance bands, 134–38
  stability ball workout, 139–47
  strength balls, 83–84
  varying, 148
Stress, 12–18
  General Adaptation Response to,
    13–17
  hormones resulting from, 14–17
  massage for reduction of, 157
Stressors, 13
Stretching:
  do's and don'ts for, 73
  importance of, 58
  for Lymph-Fit Workout, 117–18
  (*See also* Cool-down stretches)
Stroke, 59
Sugars, 178–79
Sun Salutation, 49–57, 84
  full body awareness during, 57
  full version of, 53–56
  half version of, 56–57
  for rest and renewal days, 97
  before split workouts, 109
  when traveling, 188
Swelling, 10, 11

T breather exercise, 52
Talk Test, 67
Target heart rate, 66–67
Therapeutic bath, 167
Thoracic lymph duct, 11–12
Thoracoabdominal pump, 111
Time, finding, 6–7, 28–30

Trampolines (*See also*
    Rebounders)
Traveling workouts, 185, 187–88
Turmeric, 181
Twain, Mark, 173

Uni Key Health Systems, 196

Vacation, fitness and, 189
Varying routine, 125, 148
Visualization, 185, 186, 190

Walking:
  choosing between rebounding
    and, 58
  guidelines for, 66, 69
  monitoring, 66–68
  in Phase 1, 68–70
  in Phase 2, 84
  in Phase 3, 105–6
Weight loss:
  and excess blood sugar, 168
  and liver detoxification, 4–5
  and skin/muscle tone, 32
  and sleep, 12, 168
  stress factor in, 12–18
Weight training (*See* Strength
    training)
Wescott, Wayne, 179
Workout calendar:
  Phase 1, 75–76
  Phase 2, 98–100
  Phase 3, 120–21